Hypertension

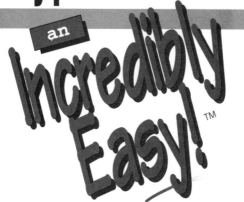

an Incredibly Easy!™

MiniGuide

Hypertension

an

Incredibly Easy!™

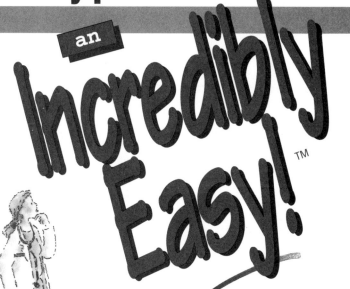

MiniGuide

Springhouse Corporation
Springhouse, Pennsylvania

Staff

Vice President
Matthew Cahill

Clinical Director
Judith A. Schilling McCann,
RN, MSN

Art Director
John Hubbard

Executive Editor
Michael Shaw

Managing Editor
Andrew T. McPhee, RN,
BSN

Clinical Editors
Pamela Mullen Kovach, RN,
BSN; Carla M. Roy, RN,
BSN, CCRN; Joan M.
Robinson, RN, MSN, CCRN;
Gwynn Sinkinson, RNC, NP

Editors
Laini Berlin, Kevin Haworth

Copy Editors
Brenna H. Mayer (manager),
Stacey Ann Follin, Pamela
Wingrod

Designers
Arlene Putterman (associate art director), Mary
Ludwicki (book designer),
Joseph John Clark, Donna
S. Morris, Susan Sheridan

Illustrator,
Bot Roda, Jacalyn B.
Facciolo

Typography
Diane Paluba (manager),
Joyce Rossi Biletz, Valerie
Molettiere

Manufacturing
Deborah Meiris (director),
Patricia K. Dorshaw (manager), Otto Mezei (book production manager)

Editorial Assistants
Beverly Lane, Marcia Mills,
Liz Schaeffer

Indexer
Barbara Hodgson

Printed in the United States of
America.

IEMHYP-010899

℞ A member of the Reed Elsevier plc group

**Library of Congress Cataloging-in
Publication Data**

Hypertension: an incredibly easy
miniguide
        p. cm.—(Miniguides)
Includes bibliographical references
and index.
        1. Hypertension Handbooks,
manuals etc. 2. Hypertension—
Nursing Handbooks, manuals, etc. I.
Springhouse Corporation. II. Series:
Incredibly easy miniguide. [DNLM:
1. Hypertension Handbooks. 2.
Hypertension Nurses' Instruction.
WG 39 H998 1999]
RC685.H8H7684 1999
616.1'32—dc21
DNLM/DLC   99-15487
ISBN 1-58255-010-7 (alk. paper)   CIP

Contents

Contributors and consultants   vi

Foreword   vii

1 Understanding hypertension   1

2 Preventing hypertension   23

3 Assessing patients with hypertension   35

4 Treating patients with hypertension   61

5 Complications   99

6 Teaching patients with hypertension   119

Index   139

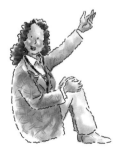

Contributors and consultants

Joanne M. Bartelmo, RN, MSN, CCRN
Clinical Educator
Pottstown (Pa.) Memorial
Medical Center

Nancy Cirone, RN,C, MSN, CDE
Director of Education
Warminster (Pa.) Hospital

Margaret Friant Cramer, RN, MSN
Clinical Supervisor
Cardiac Solutions, Inc.
Fort Washington, Pa.

Michael Carter, RN, DNSc, FAAN
Dean and Professor
College of Nursing
University of Tennessee
Memphis

Pamela Mullen Kovach, RN, BSN
Independent Clinical
Consultant
Perkiomenville, Pa.

Patricia A. Lange, RN, MSN, EdD (candidate), **CS, CCRN**
Graduate Nursing Program
Coordinator and Assistant
Professor of Nursing
Hawaii Pacific University
Kaneohe

Mary Ann Siciliano McLaughlin, RN, MSN
Clinical Supervisor
Cardiac Solutions, Inc.
Fort Washington, Pa.

Lori Musolf Neri, RN, MSN, CCRN
Clinical Instructor
Villanova (Pa.) University

Joseph L. Neri, DO, FACC
Cardiologist
The Heart Care Group
Allentown, Pa.

Robert Rauch
Manager of Government
Economics
Amgen, Inc.
Thousand Oaks, Calif.

Larry E. Simmons, RN, PhD (candidate)
Clinical Instructor
University of Missouri-
Kansas City

Foreword

Hypertension affects as many as 60 million Americans. Many patients with hypertension show no signs. As a result, elevated blood pressure is commonly revealed as part of a routine checkup. It may also remain undiscovered until it begins to damage other body systems.

Caring for a patient with hypertension requires a full understanding of the disorder and its implications for care. At once accurate, authoritative, and completely up-to-date, *Hypertension: An Incredibly Easy MiniGuide* can help you gain an in-depth understanding of hypertension in an amazingly fun and exciting way.

The first chapter, *Understanding hypertension,* lays the foundation for your understanding by providing basic facts about the pathophysiology of hypertension and the effects of hypertension on the body. The next three chapters cover prevention, assessment, and treatment for hypertension. The fifth chapter covers hypertension complications, and the final chapter covers patient teaching.

Throughout the book, you'll find features designed to make learning about hypertension lively and entertaining. For instance, *Memory joggers* provide clever tricks for remembering key points. *Checklists,* in the style of a classroom chalkboard, provide at-a-glance summaries of important facts.

Cartoon characters that nearly pop off the page provide light-hearted chuckles as well as reinforcement of essential material. And a *Quick quiz* at the end of every chapter gives you a chance to assess your learning and refresh your memory at the same time.

The depth of information contained in this truly pocket-size guide will impress even the most experienced health care professional. If you want a quick-learn, comprehensive reference about one of the most common conditions encountered in health care, I can't think of a more fitting resource than *Hypertension: An Incredibly Easy MiniGuide.* It packs a wallop.

Michael Carter, RN, DNSc, FAAN
Dean and Professor
College of Nursing
University of Tennessee
Memphis

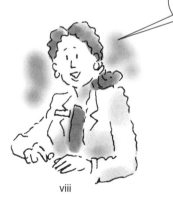

Professional development that's fun and exciting? Incredible!

Understanding hypertension

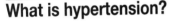

Key facts
- Hypertension can occur occasionally or be present all the time.
- The condition is classified as essential or secondary, depending on its cause.
- Malignant hypertension can arise from either form of hypertension and is a medical emergency.
- Hypertension damages blood vessels in organs such as the heart, brain, and kidneys.

What is hypertension?

Hypertension is an intermittent or sustained elevation of a person's blood pressure. This elevation may occur during the systolic phase (when the heart is at work) or during the diastolic phase (when the heart is at rest).

Generally, a sustained systolic blood pressure of 140 mm Hg or higher or a diastolic pressure of 90 mm Hg or higher, indicates hypertension. (See *Classifying blood pressure.*) Hypertension should be diagnosed on the basis of several readings taken at different times on different days and in different settings.

Hypertension, commonly known as high blood pressure, affects as many as 60 million Americans. Because a patient may have hypertension without showing symptoms, elevated blood pressure is commonly revealed as part of a routine checkup. It may also remain undiscovered until it begins to damage other body systems.

Types of hypertension

There are two main types of hypertension — essential and secondary. Malignant hypertension, a fulminant form of hypertension, can arise from essential or secondary hypertension. (See *Malignant hypertension,* page 4.)

Essence of essential hypertension

Essential hypertension, also called primary or idiopathic hypertension, accounts for 90% of all hypertension cases. Its exact cause remains unknown.

Advice from the experts

Classifying blood pressure

Blood pressure status can be classified according to six main categories, depending on systolic and diastolic readings. This chart outlines each category and the systolic and diastolic parameters for each.

Category	Systolic pressure (in mm Hg)	Diastolic pressure (in mm Hg)
Normal	Below 130	Below 85
High normal	130 to 139	85 to 89
Stage 1 (mild) hypertension	140 to 159	90 to 99
Stage 2 (moderate) hypertension	160 to 179	100 to 109
Stage 3 (severe) hypertension	180 to 209	110 to 119
Stage 4 (very severe) hypertension	210 or above	120 or above

Essential hypertension usually begins as an insidious disease, developing slowly and causing no symptoms. Without treatment, essential hypertension can become malignant and develop into a severe, fulminant disorder.

Got a second for secondary hypertension?

Secondary hypertension results from another condition, such as kidney disease or an endocrine disorder, that raises pe-

Malignant hypertension

Malignant hypertension is a medical emergency characterized by marked blood pressure elevation, papilledema, retinal hemorrhages and exudates, and manifestations of hypertensive encephalopathy, such as severe headache, vomiting, visual disturbances, transient paralysis, seizures, stupor, and coma. Heart failure and acute renal failure may also develop.

Cause

The cause of malignant hypertension is unknown, though dilation of cerebral arteries and generalized arteriolar fibrinoid necrosis contribute to the disorder.

Treatment

Emergency treatment aims to quickly reduce blood pressure and identify the underlying cause. Rapid-acting vasodilators such as nitroprusside may be used to reduce blood pressure. Loop diuretics or cardiac glycosides may be used for a patient with heart failure.

ripheral vascular resistance or cardiac output. Secondary hypertension accounts for 10% of all hypertension cases. In some instances, treating the cause cures the patient's hypertension. Some causes of secondary hypertension include:

- coarctation of the aorta
- Cushing's syndrome
- diabetes mellitus

• dysfunction of the thyroid, parathyroid, or pituitary gland
• neurologic disorders
• pheochromocytoma
• pregnancy
• primary aldosteronism
• renal parenchymal disease
• renovascular disease.

Secondary hypertension results from another condition such as kidney disease.

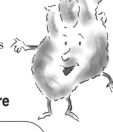

What can hypertension lead to?

If left untreated, hypertension can lead to serious complications, such as heart disease, renal failure, stroke, and death.

Understanding blood pressure

The term *blood pressure* refers to the amount of pressure that blood exerts on the arteries as it flows through them. Several elements determine a person's blood pressure, including:

Sure, blame everything on me!

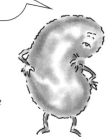

• blood volume
• capillary fluid shift
• hormonal regulators (see *Understanding the renin-angiotensin-aldosterone system,* page 6)
• neural regulators
• vascular resistance.

Understanding the renin-angiotensin-aldosterone system

The renin-angiotensin-aldosterone system plays a key role in blood pressure regulation. Here's how the system works to increase blood pressure:

• Sodium depletion, decreased blood pressure, and dehydration stimulate the release of renin.
• Renin reacts with angiotensin, converting it to angiotensin I.
• Angiotensin I becomes angiotensin II in the lungs.
• Angiotensin II constricts arterioles (raising arterial blood pressure), constricts veins (promoting venous return to the heart and increasing blood volume), and increases aldosterone secretion (retaining sodium and water).

Pressure at work

Blood volume, also known as cardiac output, refers to the amount of blood ejected each minute from the heart's left ventricle. Blood volume is the main factor in determining systolic blood pressure.

The kidneys help control blood volume by regulating sodium and water levels. Under conditions that increase heart rate or stroke volume, blood volume also increases, thus increasing systolic blood pressure.

Pressure at rest

Vascular resistance, a term referring to the amount of pressure exerted by arterial walls against the blood flowing through them, can be affected by blood viscosity and diameter of the vessel lumen or wall. Vascular resistance is the main factor that determines diastolic blood pressure.

Nervous response

Under normal conditions, neural regulators help keep blood pressure within appropriate levels. Neural regulators include baroreceptors and chemoreceptors. Baroreceptors are nerve endings embedded in blood vessels that respond to vessel wall stretching.

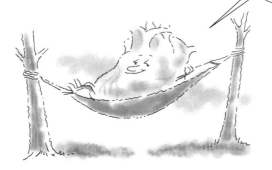

How much resistance I meet determines my diastolic blood pressure.

Chemoreceptors are nerve endings in carotid artery walls, the aorta, and the medulla. These receptors respond to low blood levels of oxygen and carbon dioxide.

Hormones help

Hormonal regulators include norepinephrine, epinephrine, renin, antidiuretic hormone, and the prostaglandins. Like neural regulators, hormonal regulators can cause changes that lead to adjustments in blood pressure.

Doin' the fluid shift

In capillary fluid shift, blood moves between vessels and extravascular spaces in response to the volume of blood in the vessels. This fluid exchange helps regulate arterial pressure.

Pathophysiology

Hypertension occurs when the body fails to regulate blood pressure properly. This lack of regulation allows the pressure to build beyond appropriate levels. Exactly why the body's internal regulating meth-

(Text continues on page 17.)

Normal blood pressure

To understand hypertension, you must first understand normal blood pressure. Blood pressure results from blood being pumped out of the heart (systolic pressure) against resistance created by arteriolar walls in peripheral blood vessels (diastolic pressure). The peripheral blood pressure of a healthy adult ranges from 95 to 140 mm Hg systolic and from 60 to 90 mm Hg diastolic. This illustration shows how ventricular contraction creates pressure within blood vessels.

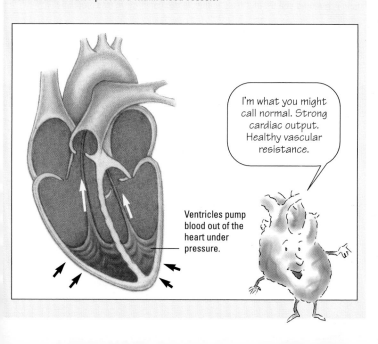

Causes of hypertension

Hypertension may result from a number of conditions, including atherosclerosis, increased blood volume or viscosity, excessive renin secretion, and stress. The illustrations on the following pages show the various causes of hypertension.

Atherosclerosis

In atherosclerosis, a plaque can obstruct the free flow of blood. As a result, blood flow is reduced and tissues distal to the obstruction receive less blood.

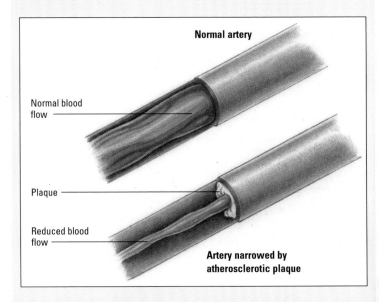

Normal artery

Normal blood flow

Plaque

Reduced blood flow

Artery narrowed by atherosclerotic plaque

Causes of hypertension *(continued)*

Effect on heart

To maintain blood flow distal to an obstruction in an artery, the heart must contract more forcefully. More forceful contractions push blood past an obstruction but may result in hypertension.

(continued)

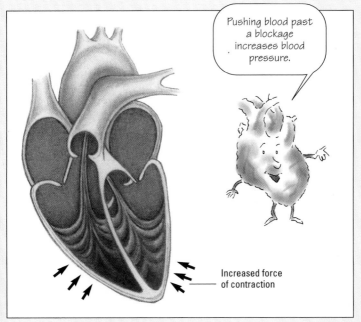

Pushing blood past a blockage increases blood pressure.

Increased force of contraction

Causes of hypertension *(continued)*

Volume and viscosity

Greater blood volume or more viscous blood places extra pressure on blood vessel walls. To push a high volume of blood or highly viscous blood into the circulation, the heart must pump more forcefully, leading to hypertension.

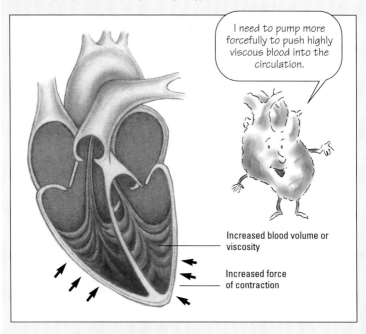

Causes of hypertension *(continued)*

Too much renin

An excessive amount of renin secreted by the kidneys can lead to hypertension. This flowchart explains the pathophysiology of excessive renin secretion. (Start reading at the bottom and, like blood pressure, work your way up.)

(continued)

Increased blood volume and vascular resistance cause hypertension.

Arteriolar constriction increases peripheral vascular resistance.

Retained sodium and water increase blood volume.

Aldosterone causes sodium and water retention.

Angiotensin II causes arteriolar constriction and aldosterone secretion.

Angiotensin I is converted to angiotensin II (a potent vasoconstrictor) in lungs.

Renin helps convert angiotensin to angiotensin I in liver.

Kidneys release renin into bloodstream.

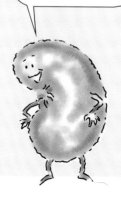

The renin-angiotensin-aldosterone system starts with me... and pretty much ends with me. Call this system the Kidney Connection.

Causes of hypertension *(continued)*

Stress

Stress can play a role in the development of hypertension. This flowchart shows the steps involved. (As in the previous flowchart, start reading at the bottom.)

Increased CO and resistance lead to hypertension.

These effects increase cardiac output (CO) and peripheral vascular resistance.

Sympathetic stimulation increases heart rate, cardiac contractility, and vasoconstriction.

Stress stimulates sympathetic nervous system.

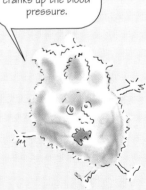

See what stress does? It really cranks up the blood pressure.

Effects of sustained hypertension

Sustained hypertension can damage blood vessels. Vascular injury begins with alternating areas of dilation and constriction in the arterioles. The illustrations below show how blood vessel damage occurs from sustained hypertension.

(continued)

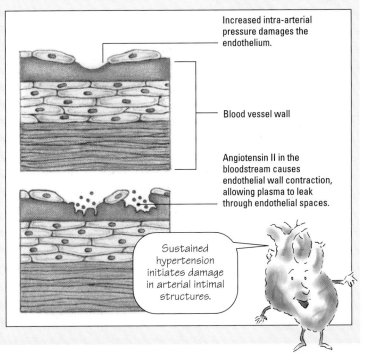

Increased intra-arterial pressure damages the endothelium.

Blood vessel wall

Angiotensin II in the bloodstream causes endothelial wall contraction, allowing plasma to leak through endothelial spaces.

Sustained hypertension initiates damage in arterial intimal structures.

Effects of sustained hypertension *(continued)*

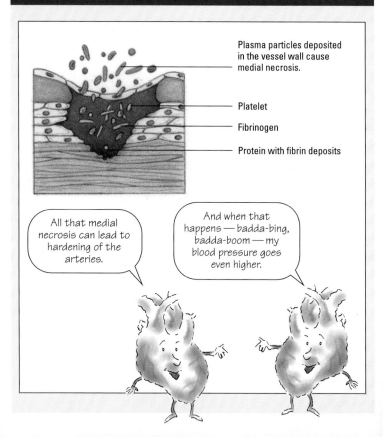

ods fail remains unknown, though several theories exist.

Essential hypertension

Essential hypertension may arise from:
• increased blood volume resulting from renal or hormonal dysfunction
• changes in the arteriolar bed, which leads to increased vascular resistance and higher blood pressure
• abnormally increased tone in the sensory nervous system, which causes increased peripheral vascular resistance
• increased arteriolar thickening (caused by genetic factors) that leads to increased peripheral vascular resistance and higher blood pressure
• abnormal renin release resulting in the formation of angiotensin II, which constricts arterioles and increases blood volume, thereby increasing blood pressure.

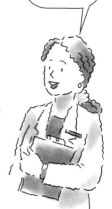

In patients with hypertension, the body's pressure-regulating mechanisms fail.

Secondary hypertension

With secondary hypertension, blood pressure increases due to changes caused by an underlying condition. (See *How secondary hypertension develops,* pages 18 and 19.) The mechanism be-

(Text continues on page 20.)

Now I get it!

How secondary hypertension develops

Secondary hypertension develops as a result of an underlying condition and occurs most commonly in children. This table describes the the main causes of secondary hypertension and their effects.

Cause	Effects
Coarctation of the aorta	A narrowing of the aorta leads to decreased blood supply in the legs. While the heart works harder to increase the supply, blood pressure rises in the upper part of the body.
Cushing's syndrome	Increased cortisol levels raise blood pressure by increasing renal sodium retention, angiotensin II levels, and vascular response to norepinephrine.
Diabetes mellitus	Increased blood glucose levels increase athero-sclerosis in the blood vessels. The resulting narrowing and leaking of the vessels can cause an increase in blood pressure.
Dysfunction of the parathyroid gland	Dysfunction of the parathyroid gland can lead to a calcium imbalance, affecting smooth-muscle contractions and causing vasoconstriction.
Dysfunction of the pituitary gland	Dysfunction of the pituitary gland can cause too much thyroid-stimulating hormone to be produced, leading to hyperthyroidism, which, in turn, increases blood pressure.
Dysfunction of the thyroid gland	Dysfunction of the thyroid gland produces too much thyroid hormone, which speeds up the heart and increases blood pressure.

How secondary hypertension develops *(continued)*

Cause	Effects
Neurologic disorders	Autonomic hyperreflexia in a patient with a spinal cord injury can result in episodic hypertension. In addition, various tumors can stimulate excessive release of catecholamines, causing hypertension.
Pheochromo-cytoma	Adrenal medulla tumor increases secretion of epinephrine (increases cardiac contractility and rate) and norepinephrine (increases peripheral vascular resistance).
Pregnancy	Although the cause remains unknown, vasospasm causing arteriolar constriction and increased peripheral vascular resistance raises blood pressure, usually after the 20th week of gestation.
Primary aldosteronism	Increased intravascular volume, altered sodium concentrations in vessel walls, or very high aldosterone levels cause vasoconstriction.
Renal parenchymal disease	Chronic glomerulonephritis or pyelonephritis causes inflammatory changes in the kidneys, which interfere with sodium excretion. This stimulates the renin-angiotensin-aldosterone system, causing blood pressure to rise.
Renovascular disease	Renal artery stenosis caused by atherosclerosis or abnormalities of the arterial wall leads to reduced kidney perfusion. This stimulates the renin-angiotensin-aldosterone system, causing blood pressure to rise.

hind the increase in blood pressure
varies according to the underlying cause.

Quick quiz

1. The most common type of hypertension is:

    A.   essential.

    B.   malignant.

    C.   secondary.

Answer: A. Of all patients with hypertension, 90% have essential hypertension, also known as primary or idiopathic hypertension.

2. Secondary hypertension is a result of an underlying condition, such as:

    A.   coarctation of the aorta.

    B.   human immunodeficiency virus infection.

    C.   peritonitis.

Answer: A. Secondary hypertension derives from an underlying condition, such as pregnancy or coarctation of the aorta, both of which raise peripheral vascular resistance.

3. Endothelial damage in the blood vessels of a patient with hypertension is typically the result of increased:

    A.   extravascular pressure.

    B.   interstitial pressure.

    C.   intra-arterial pressure.

Answer: C. Increased intra-arterial pressure begins weakening the endothelial wall, allowing plasma leakage, deposition of plasma constituents in the vessel wall, and development of medial necrosis.

4. Abnormal renin release results in the formation of angiotensin II, which:

    A.   dilates arterioles and lowers blood volume.

    B.   constricts arterioles and increases blood volume.

    C.   constricts arterioles and lowers blood volume.

Answer: B. Abnormal renin release results in the formation of angiotensin II, which constricts arterioles and increases blood volume, thereby increasing blood pressure.

Scoring

★★★ If you answered all four questions correctly, dy-no-mite! You've mastered the ups and downs of systole — and diastole too, for that matter!

★★ If you answered three questions correctly, coolness! You're handling the (blood) pressure like a pro!

★ If you answered fewer than three questions correctly, lighten up! When the pressure's off, you'll come bouncing back in no time!

2

Preventing hypertension

Key facts
- ◆ Hypertension affects significantly more blacks than whites.
- ◆ Modifying risk factors can reduce the risk of essential hypertension.
- ◆ Even borderline systolic hypertension increases the risk of developing organ damage.

Identifying risk factors

Hypertension afflicts more than 60 million adults. Blacks are particularly at risk; they develop hypertension at twice the rate of whites. In addition, a black person with hypertension is four times as likely as a white person to die of complications of the disorder.

You may face a significant risk of hypertension.

The good news

Health care professionals are making progress in the battle against hypertension. The Centers for Disease Control and Prevention reports that:

• Only 2 out of 10 Americans have blood pressure above 140/90 mm Hg, indicating a greater than 10% decline in hypertension over the past 20 years.

• Three out of four people with hypertension are aware of their condition. More than half of them receive regular treatment for hypertension.

• About 30% of people with hypertension successfully control their blood pressure.

The bad news

Despite these gains, hypertension still poses significant risks. New studies warn that even people with borderline isolated systolic hypertension (up to 159/90 mm Hg) face potentially serious complications, including:

• 31% higher risk of myocardial infarction

• 95% higher risk of cerebrovascular accident

• 43% higher death rate overall, when compared with patients whose blood pressure is under 140/90 mm Hg.

Risky business

Several nonmodifiable risk factors appear to predispose a patient to hypertension. Although these risk factors can't be changed, early identification can help catch hypertension before it develops or at an early stage.

Nonmodifiable risk factors include age, family history, gender, and race.

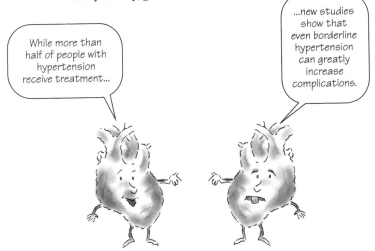

While more than half of people with hypertension receive treatment...

...new studies show that even borderline hypertension can greatly increase complications.

Advancing age

Several age-related changes may contribute to the development of hypertension, including decreased glomerular filtration rate, reduced baroreceptor sensitivity and, the most significant, atherosclerosis. Atherosclerosis can:
- increase the rigidity of the aortic wall
- increase the rigidity of peripheral arteries
- lead to a rise in systemic vascular resistance and blood pressure.

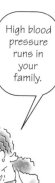

High blood pressure runs in your family.

It's all in the family

Hypertension appears to fall under genetic influences. A person with family members who have a history of hypertension faces significantly increased risk of developing the disorder.

About that gender issue

Although men and women face approximately equal risk of developing hypertension, some gender-specific factors may contribute to increased risk. For example, the use of oral contraceptives has been associated with hypertension. Researchers think oral contraceptive use activates the renin-angiotensin-aldosterone system and causes blood pressure to rise.

Hypertension and race

Blacks have twice the hypertension risk of whites. Furthermore, the disease commonly develops earlier in blacks, takes a more severe course, and causes more deaths at a younger age.

Prevention strategies

In most cases, the exact cause of a person's hypertension remains unknown. However, many patients exhibit risk factors that, if modified, can substantially reduce their risk of hypertension. These modifiable risk factors include:
- being overweight
- high-fat diet
- lack of exercise
- smoking
- stress.

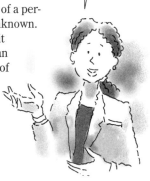

To catch hypertension early, monitor blood pressure regularly — at least once a year.

Slim down the pressure

Overweight patients face significant increased risk of hypertension, but weight loss can be an effective tool in preventing the condition. By reducing weight, a patient can reduce his blood pressure substantially, even if he doesn't reach his ideal body weight. Weight reduction also lessens the heart's workload, increasing overall cardiac health.

Patients in early adulthood need to be even more aware of their weight. Obesity that occurs in a person between ages 20 and 30 is a significant risk factor for subsequent hypertension.

Less salt, more bananas

Diet changes for preventing hypertension should focus on restricting sodium and increasing potassium intake. (See *Meeting daily requirements,* pages 30 and 31.) Moderate sodium restriction — 2 g or less per day — can enhance diuretic therapy and reduce potassium loss.

Preliminary evidence also suggests that increased potassium intake, independent of decreased sodium intake, helps lower blood pressure.

Sources of potassium
- Bananas
- Orange juice
- Tomatoes
- Sweet potatoes
- Lean pork or veal
- Low-fat milk or yogurt
- Catfish, cod, or flounder
- Dry peas and beans

Patients should also reduce daily alcohol and caffeine consumption. Excessive alcohol use may progressively increase systolic and diastolic pressure. Caffeine can have a vasoconstricting effect that could raise blood pressure.

Reducing dietary fat, especially saturated fat, can help lower blood pressure by helping reduce weight.

A banana a day can help lower blood pressure. And they taste yummy!

Advice from the experts

Meeting daily requirements

Meeting daily recommended requirements of certain vitamins and minerals, such as calcium and magnesium, may help reduce the risk of hypertension.

Eat your broccoli

Studies have shown that many people with low-calcium diets have high blood pressure. Some researchers theorize that defective vascular metabolism, stemming from insufficient calcium in the diet, underlies the abnormal vasoconstriction that occurs in patients with hypertension. To maintain good health, adults should develop a diet that meets the recommended requirements of calcium, at least 800 mg/day. Sources of calcium, in descending order of the amount of calcium contained in each food, include:

- tofu
- low-fat cheese
- low-fat milk or yogurt
- broccoli
- collard greens.

Eating like a squirrel

A low-magnesium diet may increase blood pressure. Magnesium is important for nerve impulse transmission and muscle contraction. The patient with hypertension may need to modify his diet to reach his daily requirement of 400 mg of magnesium. Sources of magnesium include:

- dry peas and beans
- green leafy vegetables
- nuts and seeds
- whole grains.

Meeting daily requirements *(continued)*

Something is fishy here

Eating large amounts of omega-3 fatty acids, found in such fish as mackerel and salmon, may help reduce hypertension. Taking fish oil supplements is unwise because high doses of the oil can cause adverse effects. Because supplements are also high in calories and fat, encourage patients to include low-fat fish dishes in their diet instead.

Walk, jog, or swim

Regular isotonic exercise — such as walking, jogging, or swimming — may help reduce blood pressure and contribute to weight loss. Warn the patient to start his exercise program gradually,

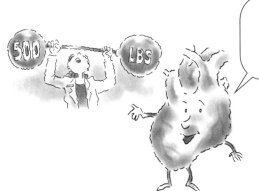

Advice from the experts

Stress connection

Some people believe that stress predisposes a person to hypertension. Although acute physical or emotional stress may elevate blood pressure briefly, a direct relationship has never been proved between stress and essential hypertension.

after medical evaluation, and to avoid isometric exercises such as weight lifting that greatly raise blood pressure.

Support for stopping

Nicotine, a vasoconstrictor, can increase blood pressure. Encourage smoking cessation through support groups, chewing gum with nicotine in it, nicotine transdermal systems, or a non-nicotine smoking cessation aid such as bupropion hydrochloride.

Takin' it easy

Reducing stress can help the patient lower his metabolic rate, thus increasing cardiac health. (See *Stress connection*.) Implement techniques to reduce your patient's stress level. Discuss the following topics with the patient:

• biofeedback

• relaxation techniques, such as deep breathing, progressive muscle relaxation, and visualization

• sources of stress

• ways to minimize or eliminate stress

• strategies for coping with unavoidable stress.

Quick quiz

1. Researchers think that oral contraceptive use leads to hypertension because these drugs:

    A. activate the renin-angiotensin-aldosterone system.

    B. increase the levels of circulating estrogen.

    C. reduce the excretion rate of sodium and potassium.

Answer: A. Researchers theorize that oral contraceptives activate the renin-angiotensin-aldosterone system, thus causing blood pressure to rise.

2. Moderate sodium restriction (2 g or less per day) can reduce:

    A. potassium loss.

    B. peripheral vascular resistance.

    C. the risk of stroke.

Answer: A. Moderate sodium restriction can enhance diuretic therapy and reduce potassium loss.

3. Smoking should be avoided for a person with hypertension because nicotine acts as a:

    A. vasoconstrictor.

    B. vasodilator.

    C. vasospastic drug.

Answer: A. Smoking should be avoided for a person with hypertension because nicotine acts as a vasoconstrictor.

Scoring

☆☆☆   If you answered all three questions correctly, perfect! You've earned a P for Prevention!

☆☆   If you answered two questions correctly, right on! Reducing risk clearly rivets your attention!

☆   If you answered fewer than two questions correctly, try not to worry. Who needs all that stress? Not us!

3

Assessing patients with hypertension

Key facts
- ◆ Many patients with hypertension remain asymptomatic and may be unaware of their condition.
- ◆ Diagnosing hypertension depends on accurate and repeated blood pressure measurements.
- ◆ After hypertension has been diagnosed, assessment should focus on identifying signs of organ damage.

When you suspect hypertension

In many cases, hypertension is asymptomatic, especially in its early stages. You may discover hypertension in a patient only incidentally, while evaluating another disorder or during a routine blood pressure screening program.

As hypertension becomes severe, it can produce various signs and symptoms.

Cerebrovascular

Cerebrovascular signs and symptoms of hypertension include:
- blackouts
- blurred vision
- dizziness
- headache (see *Hypertension headaches*)
- one-sided numbness or weakness
- syncope.

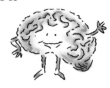

Cardiovascular

Cardiovascular signs and symptoms of hypertension include:
- chest pain
- dyspnea
- palpitations
- peripheral edema.

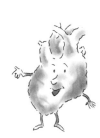

Still more signs and symptoms

Other signs and symptoms of hypertension include:
- excess urinary sediment
- fatigue
- nocturia
- nosebleed
- peripheral edema
- weakness.

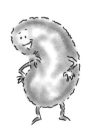

Warning!

Hypertension headaches

Headaches caused by hypertension typically occur in the occipital area and worsen as the patient wakes up in the morning. A tension headache, in comparison, usually occurs in the frontal area and worsens during the day. Blood pressure usually must increase markedly before causing a headache.

Taking a health history

Your approach to taking a patient's history depends on whether your patient has known hypertension. If you suspect hypertension:

• focus on confirming the diagnosis

• determine the disorder's origin — essential hypertension or hypertension that derives from another condition

• identify whether organ damage has occurred.

For a newbie...

Keep in mind that a patient previously unaware of his hypertension may seek medical care either for an unrelated

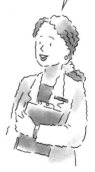

If you suspect hypertension, focus on confirming the diagnosis and identifying organ damage.

problem or for hypertension-related symptoms. If the patient has newly discovered hypertension, ask questions about:

- related symptoms
- how long he has had each symptom
- how the symptom affects his daily routine
- whether he has had other associated symptoms.

In case of pain...

If the patient is suffering pain, ask about:

- location of the pain
- duration of the pain
- whether the pain radiates
- intensity of the pain
- precipitating factors
- exacerbating factors
- relieving factors.

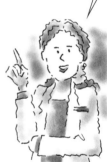

Check if the patient's symptoms of high blood pressure affect his daily routine.

When hypertension already exists...

If the patient has a history of hypertension, ask questions concerning:

- his compliance with therapy
- therapeutic effectiveness
- associated symptoms.

Medical history

For a patient with newly discovered hypertension, ask questions about:
- prior symptoms, if any
- his last doctor's visit, prior medical diagnoses, and treatment
- major acute or chronic illnesses requiring hospitalization
- use of alcohol, tobacco, or caffeine
- prescription, over-the-counter, or recreational drugs
- allergies to foods, drugs, or other agents
- pregnancies, menopause, or use of oral contraceptives or estrogens (for a female)
- cardiovascular risk factors
- renal damage
- obesity.

Family history

Ask questions about blood relatives who have had:
- diabetes mellitus
- heart disease
- hypertension
- kidney disease
- stroke.

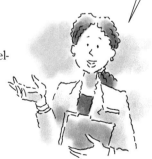

For a patient with a history of hypertension, find out if he's sticking to his treatment regimen.

Social history

To gather a social history, ask about the patient's:
- daily activities
- diet
- educational background
- exercise habits
- family relationships
- living arrangements
- occupation
- sexual function
- sleep habits.

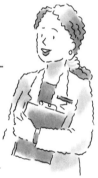

Ask about a family history of hypertension or heart disease.

Examining a patient with hypertension

A thorough physical assessment can help alert you to a patient who might have undiagnosed hypertension. For a patient with known hypertension, a physical examination may reveal hypertension's effects on the body.

Inspection

Inspection of a person with hypertension may reveal:
- peripheral edema, in late stages when heart failure is present

• café-au-lait spots on skin (common with pheochromocytoma)
• retinal blood vessel damage, found through funduscopic examination. (See *Retinal funduscopic examination,* page 42.)

Palpation

Palpation of a patient with hypertension may reveal:
• pulsating abdominal mass, suggesting an abdominal aneurysm
• carotid artery stenosis or occlusion
• enlarged kidneys, indicating polycystic disease, a cause of secondary hypertension
• enlarged thyroid gland
• skin temperature changes
• weak or absent pulses.

Auscultation

Auscultation of a patient with hypertension may reveal:
• carotid bruit
• systolic or diastolic pressure, both of which may be elevated
• increase in diastolic pressure when moving from a supine to a standing position, suggesting essential hypertension

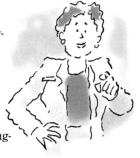

Retinal damage found on funduscopic examination may indicate hypertension.

Peak technique

Retinal funduscopic examination

Examination of the retina — the only site where arteries can be seen without invasive techniques — provides a reliable indicator of the severity of hypertension. Damage can be assessed on a scale of four grades, shown here.

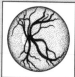

Grade I: mild sclerosis or arteriolar narrowing, associated with mildly elevated blood pressure

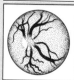

Grade II: marked retinal changes with increased light reflexes and vein compression at crossings, which indicates progressive, sustained hypertension

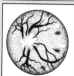

Grade III: angiospastic retinitis and sclerotic arteriolar changes, possibly with edema, which indicates severe, sustained hypertension, possibly associated with evidence of cardiac or renal complications

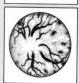

Grade IV: papilledema with exudates and extensive hemorrhages, disk edema, and severe arteriolar narrowing with diffuse retinitis, which indicates malignant hypertension

• decrease in diastolic blood pressure when moving from a supine to a standing position, possibly indicating secondary hypertension
• abdominal bruit heard just to the right or left of the umbilicus or in the flanks, if renal artery stenosis is present
• bruits over the abdominal aorta, femoral arteries, and carotid artery
• murmurs or third or fourth heart sounds, which may indicate left ventricle hypertrophy or early heart failure
• wheezes or crackles in the lungs, which may indicate heart failure.

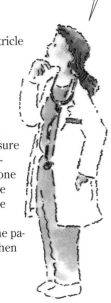

If blood pressure falls when the patient stands up, he may have secondary hypertension.

Measuring blood pressure

In most cases, hypertension is diagnosed through repeated blood pressure measurements, which are then compared to average readings for someone of that patient's age and gender. (See *Average blood pressure readings*, page 44.) To ensure accurate blood pressure measurement, consider how the patient is positioned and where and when you take the readings.

Advice from the experts

Average blood pressure readings

Average blood pressure readings vary by age. This chart outlines ages and the average blood pressure for each.

Age in years	Average reading
4	98/60
6	105/60
10	112/64
11 to 20	120/75
21 to 30	124/78
31 to 40	126/80
41 to 50	130/82
51 to 60	138/84
61 to 70	140/82 (male); 152/84 (female)
71 to 80	142/80 (male); 156/82 (female)
over 80	142/78 (male); 140/89 (female)

Keeping the patient's arm supported at heart level ensures an accurate reading.

At heart level

Seat your patient comfortably, with his arm slightly flexed and his forearm supported at heart level on a smooth surface. Blood pressure rises with the arm below heart level and drops with the arm above heart level — in

both cases by as much as 10 mm Hg.
(See *Position pointers*, page 46.)

For the initial examination, measure
and record the blood pressure in both
arms. For subsequent examinations, use
the arm with the higher initial pressure.

Comfort = accuracy

To ensure accurate results, take blood
pressure in a quiet room at a comfortable
temperature. Because anxiety, food intake, tobacco use, bladder distention,
pain, and talking can affect blood pressure, try to control or eliminate these
stimuli during measurement.

If possible, instruct the patient to avoid
exposure to cold, exertion, smoking, and
eating for 30 minutes before measurement and to avoid postural changes for 5
minutes beforehand. In addition, make
sure that clothing or other material isn't
constricting his arm.

Correct cuffs

Use the correct cuff width for your patient's arm. If the bladder of the cuff is
too narrow, the reading will be falsely
high. If it's too wide, the reading will be

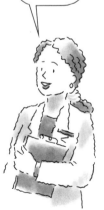

For
accurate
results,
measure
blood
pressure
when the
patient is
relaxed.

Position pointers

When measuring blood pressure, the position of the patient and the blood pressure cuff can affect accuracy of the reading. Position the patient and the blood pressure cuff as follows:

• Have the patient sit in a chair with his back supported, both feet comfortably on the floor. Sitting on the side of a bed or examining table can raise blood pressure by up to 10 mm Hg.

• Make sure the patient's arm is resting at heart level. If the arm hangs at the side, blood pressure can rise 8 mm Hg.

• Take the blood pressure in a quiet, warm setting. A noisy or cold environment could raise blood pressure.

• Wrap the cuff snugly around the upper arm above the antecubital area.

• Place the lower border of the cuff about 1" (2.5 cm) above the antecubital space.

• Place the bell of the stethoscope on the brachial artery at the point where you hear the strongest beats.

falsely low. The bladder width should be 40% of the circumference of the patient's arm at midpoint (or 20% wider than the arm's diameter).

The bladder length also affects measurement accuracy. Make sure the length is approximately twice the recommended width.

Now we're ready

Palpate the brachial artery and place the stethoscope's bell over it firmly so that its complete circumference touches the skin. (See *Positioning the cuff and stethoscope,* page 48.) The bell is used because it amplifies low-frequency sounds better than the diaphragm.

With the stethoscope in place, close the pump valve and pump up the cuff bladder until the pressure is about 30 mm Hg above the point at which the pulse disappears. Release the pressure at a rate of 2 to 3 mm Hg/second.

Listening for the Korotkoff symphony

With the stethoscope's bell over the brachial artery, listen for Korotkoff's sounds, produced by blood movement and vessel vibration. Some patients, however, might have an auscultatory gap that can affect readings. (See *Bridging the auscultatory gap,* page 49.) As the cuff pressure declines, listen for these phases of blood pressure:

• *phase I* — marked by the first faint, clear, tapping sounds of gradually increasing intensity

Positioning the cuff and stethoscope

Make sure to position the blood pressure cuff and bell of the stethoscope properly when measuring blood pressure. This illustration shows the proper placement for measuring a blood pressure.

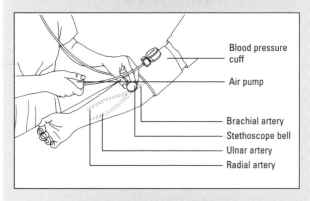

- *phase II* — marked by a murmur or swishing sound
- *phase III* — marked by increased sound intensity and crispness
- *phase IV* — marked by distinct, abrupt muffling of sounds that gives them a soft, blowing quality

Peak technique

Bridging the auscultatory gap

You may hear an auscultatory gap in some hypertensive patients. An auscultatory gap is the premature, temporary disappearance of sounds late in phases I and II. Sounds disappear as pressure drops and reappear at a lower pressure level.

Because an auscultatory gap may cover a range of up to 40 mm Hg, you may seriously underestimate systolic pressure or overestimate diastolic pressure unless you exclude the gap by first palpating for disappearance of the radial pulse as you increase cuff presence.

- *phase V* — marked by disappearance of sounds.

In the fifth movement — er, phase — of the Korotkoff symphony, sounds disappear.

Write this down

Record systolic pressure as the point at which you hear the initial tapping sound (phase I). Record the diastolic pressure as the point at which sounds disappear (phase V).

When the arm's unavailable

In some circumstances, you may need to measure blood pressure in another extremity. Use the thigh instead of the arm, and use a larger, wider cuff. Expect the thigh's systolic pressure to exceed the arm's by 10 to 30 mm Hg. The diastolic pressure remains essentially the same.

You may also measure blood pressure using an automatic monitor. (See *Automatic blood pressure monitoring,* pages 52 and 53.)

Diagnostic tests

A number of tests can help identify predisposing risk factors for hypertension and help determine the condition's cause. These tests include:
• chest X-ray, which may demonstrate evidence of cardiomegaly
• renal ultrasound, which may reveal renal atrophy
• renal flow scan, which may reveal abnormalities of blood flow indicative of renal artery stenosis

- electrocardiogram (ECG), which may show left ventricular hypertrophy or ischemia
- urinalysis, which may show protein, red blood cells, or white blood cells (suggesting renal disease), or glucose (suggesting diabetes)
- serum potassium level, which, if less than 3.5 mEq/L, may indicate adrenal dysfunction (primary aldosteronism)
- blood urea nitrogen level, which, if above 20 mg/dl, suggests renal disease
- serum creatinine level, which, if above 1.5 mg/dl, suggests renal disease.

An ECG and chest X-ray can help determine whether hypertension has caused heart damage.

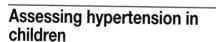

Assessing hypertension in children

When providing care for any child older than age 3, make sure to measure his blood pressure annually. Hypertension can occur in children, and early detection helps minimize the risks and ensure appropriate treatment.

(Text continues on page 54.)

Running smoothly

Automatic blood pressure monitoring

For a patient who needs frequent blood pressure measurements, use an automatic blood pressure monitor. Automatic blood pressure monitors come in several varieties, including those for ambulatory and nonambulatory patients.

For a nonambulatory patient

A continuous automatic blood pressure monitor used for a nonambulatory patient (shown below) measures:
• mean arterial pressure (MAP)
• heart rate and minutes elapsed since the last inflation
• systolic and diastolic arterial pressure.

In addition to air hoses and a pressure cuff, these monitors also have:
• switches for setting the time interval between cuff inflation
• a switch for an immediate blood pressure reading
• a switch for setting high and low MAP alarm limits.

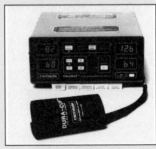

Dinamap electronic vital signs monitor

Automatic blood pressure monitoring *(continued)*

Using a continuous automatic blood pressure monitor

To use a continuous automatic blood pressure monitor, apply the blood pressure cuff as you would for a manual reading. Then turn on the machine and set the MAP limits and time interval between cuff inflation.

Troubleshooting

A change in the patient's position from one reading to another can affect readings. Try to keep the patient in the same position for each reading. To maintain consistency with blood pressure measurements, you should also:

• check cuff position periodically.

• use the proper-sized cuff.

• always use the same arm when you take manual blood pressure measurements to double-check monitor accuracy.

For an ambulatory patient

A continuous automatic blood pressure monitor used for an ambulatory patient permits you to assess your patient's blood pressure fluctuations as he performs his daily activities. In addition to a blood pressure cuff, the system includes:

• a lightweight, portable monitor that contains a microprocessor to record blood pressure measurements

• a data pack to store measurements

• a portable operating system for home analysis

• an analysis station for hospital analysis

• a detachable battery pack.

A stylish accessory

To use one of these monitors, the patient attaches the monitor to his belt or shoulder strap and slips the blood pressure cuff in place. The microprocessor records the patient's blood pressure at 6- to 60-minute intervals, depending on the medical order. After the prescribed monitoring period (usually 24 hours), blood pressure readings can be evaluated for trends, plotted on a graph, and printed out.

Use a pediatric blood pressure grid to help determine the appropriate percentile based on the child's blood pressure, age, and gender. (See *Measuring pediatric blood pressure*.) A child with blood pressure above the 95th percentile for his age and gender on three separate measurements needs further evaluation.

Measuring a child's blood pressure

For auscultatory blood pressure measurement on a child, use either the largest cuff that snugly fits the child's arm or a cuff with a bladder that's 40% of arm circumference. The inflatable bladder within the cuff should completely or nearly encircle the arm.

Muffled sounds stick around

Use the same auscultatory technique suggested for adults when measuring children. However, record diastolic pressure as the onset of muffling (phase IV), rather than the disappearance of sounds (phase V). In a child, the sounds may not disappear.

Advice from the experts

Measuring pediatric blood pressure

Each child older than age 3 should have his blood pressure checked at least once each year. The pediatric blood pressure grids shown here will help you determine the appropriate percentile based on the child's age and gender.

To use the grid, record the average systolic and diastolic pressure readings on three separate occasions. Plot the systolic measurement by age on the graph appropriate for the child's gender. Then read across to the right to find the percentile. Repeat for the diastolic pressure.

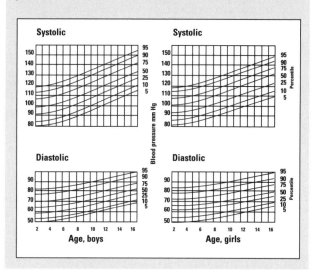

If you can't hear...

In some infants, auscultatory sounds may be too faint to hear. If you can't obtain an auscultatory blood pressure, use an ultrasonic device such as a Doppler device, which accurately measures systolic pressure.

> If you can't hear Korotkoff's sounds on an infant, use an ultrasonic device.

Palpating a blood pressure

If you don't have a Doppler device, palpation may be used to measure blood pressure. To palpate the blood pressure, place one finger over the brachial or radial artery. Inflate the cuff until the pulse is obliterated. Then slowly deflate the cuff until you feel the pulse.

Document this point as the palpable systolic blood pressure. No diastolic pressure can be obtained using this method.

Taking a child's health history

Take a thorough family history and assess the patient for other cardiovascular risks. Ask the child and his family about signs or symptoms that the child might have experienced.

What to look for

Many asymptomatic children and adolescents with elevated blood pressure:

- are overweight
- have a family history of hypertension
- usually have primary hypertension.

Symptomatic children and adolescents with elevated blood pressure typically:

- have severe hypertension with an identifiable cause
- need to be evaluated for secondary hypertension.

No drugs at first

For hypertensive children, promote nonpharmacologic therapies for initial therapy. Nonpharmacologic therapies include:

- exercise
- sodium restriction
- weight control.

Step up to the stepped care approach

If pharmacologic therapy is used for children, expect the primary care provider to use the stepped-care approach, with emphasis on minimal doses of appropriate drugs. In a stepped-care approach, mild antihypertensive drugs are used first. If they don't control blood pressure, stronger drugs are used, and so forth until the blood pressure is controlled.

Quick quiz

1. Headaches that could indicate severe hypertension occur in the:

    A.   frontal region.

    B.   occipital region.

    C.   temporal region.

Answer: B. An occipital headache that worsens in the morning can indicate severe hypertension.

2. If the bladder of a blood pressure cuff is too narrow, the reading will be:

    A.   falsely high.

    B.   falsely low.

    C.   undetectable.

Answer: A. If the bladder of the cuff is too narrow, the reading will be falsely high.

3. Phase IV of a blood pressure reading is marked by:

    A.   a murmur or swishing sound.

    B.   disappearance of the sound.

    C.   distinct, abrupt muffling of sounds.

Answer: C. Phase IV is marked by distinct, abrupt muffling of sounds that have a soft, blowing quality.

4. An auscultatory gap is a premature disappearance of sounds late in phases:
    A. I and II.
    B. II and III.
    C. III and IV.
Answer: A. An auscultatory gap is a premature disappearance of sounds late in phases I and II. Sounds disappear as pressure drops and reappear at a lower pressure level.

5. For auscultatory blood pressure measurement on a child, use either the largest cuff that snugly fits the child's arm or a cuff with a bladder that measures:
    A. 30% of arm circumference.
    B. 40% of arm circumference.
    C. 50% of arm circumference.
Answer: B. For auscultatory blood pressure measurement on a child, use either the largest cuff that snugly fits the child's arm or a cuff with a bladder that measures 40% of arm circumference, so the cuff completely or nearly encircles the arm.

Scoring

☆☆☆ If you answered all five questions correctly, all right! All's well that assesses well.

☆☆ If you answered three or four questions correctly, congratulations! Your assessment readings fall well into the normal range.

☆ If you answered fewer than three questions correctly, relax. Relaxation helps when measuring blood pressure *and* taking quizzes.

4

Treating patients with hypertension

Key facts

♦ Treatment for hypertension depends on the severity of the condition and on the presence of complications or other risk factors.

♦ Treatment can include lifestyle changes, drugs, or a combination.

♦ A number of drugs are available to reduce blood pressure, including diuretics, vasodilators, and calcium channel blockers, among others.

♦ Some patients require therapy using more than one antihypertensive drug.

Treatment overview

Treatment for hypertension generally follows a four-step process. The initial step, for patients with mild hypertension, involves lifestyle changes. If lifestyle changes fail to reduce the patient's blood pressure to acceptable levels, drugs are slowly added to the therapy regimen, and the patient's progress is monitored at

Antihypertensives and the elderly

Elderly patients commonly experience adverse drug reactions. If the adverse reaction is misinterpreted as a new medical condition, the primary care provider may prescribe a new drug to treat the new "condition."

For example, if a high dose of a nonsteroidal anti-inflammatory drug increases the blood pressure in a patient with hypertension, the primary care provider might treat this adverse reaction by changing the patient's antihypertensive medication or increasing its dosage.

Overmedication

To avoid overmedication, the primary care provider and nurse should review the elderly patient's use of prescription and over-the-counter drugs and consider their effects on blood pressure.

each step. (See *Antihypertensives and the elderly.*)

Step 1: Lifestyle changes

In step 1, the patient makes whatever lifestyle changes are indicated. These changes might include:

- exercising regularly
- losing weight
- quitting smoking
- reducing alcohol intake
- reducing stress

• avoiding added salt in his diet
• decreasing cholesterol and saturated fat in his diet.

Step 2: Single-drug therapy

If lifestyle modifications fail to reduce blood pressure, the patient will begin therapy using a single drug, usually a diuretic or beta-adrenergic blocker. (See *Drug therapy,* pages 65 to 93.) Keep in mind that if the patient has an underlying medical problem that precludes use of a diuretic or beta blocker, alternative drugs might be used, such as:
• alpha-adrenergic blockers
• angiotensin-converting enzyme (ACE) inhibitors
• calcium channel blockers
• centrally acting antiadrenergics
• vasodilators.

> Patients who need drug therapy usually start off with a diuretic or beta blocker.

Step 3: Substitute, increase, or add

If the patient complies with therapy but shows no significant improvement within 3 months, three options exist for modifying his treatment:
• substituting another drug (sequential monotherapy)

> **Hypertensive classes**
> ACE inhibitors
> Alpha-adrenergic blockers
> Beta-adrenergic blockers
> Calcium channel blockers
> Centrally acting anti-adrenergics
> Diuretics
> Vasodilators

• increasing the drug dosage (titration)
• adding a second drug from a different class of drugs (step-wise combination therapy).

Step 4: Multidrug therapy

Although some patients respond adequately to therapy with a single drug, many need a second or third drug to significantly reduce their blood pressure. In step 4, the patient begins taking two or three antihypertensive drugs in addition to a diuretic.

Step down

After about a year of successful blood pressure control, some patients can

(Text continues on page 93.)

Drug therapy

Several types of drugs for hypertension are available. They're categorized by the actions they take to reduce blood pressure and include angiotensin-converting enzyme (ACE) inhibitors, alpha and beta adrenergic blockers, calcium channel blockers, centrally acting anti-adrenergics, diuretics, and vasodilators. This section examines properties of each class as well as common adverse reactions and key special considerations for selected members of the class.

ACE inhibitors

Some drugs inhibit the effects of angiotensin II, an enzyme that constricts blood vessels and is commonly overproduced in patients with hypertension. These drugs — called ACE inhibitors — prevent angiotensin I from converting to angiotensin II. These drugs also decrease aldosterone, thus decreasing sodium and water retention. This helps patients who also have heart failure. Benazepril hydrochloride (Lotensin) is an example of an ACE inhibitor.

A similar class of the drugs, called angiotensin II blockers, prevent angiotensin II from binding to its receptors, thus preventing the blood vessel response that leads to hypertension. Losartan potassium (Cozaar) is an example of an angiotensin II blocker.

benazepril hydrochloride
Trade name: Lotensin

Adverse reactions
Common adverse reactions include angioedema; dry, persistent, nonproductive cough; fatigue; headache; hyperkalemia; and symptomatic hypotension.

Special considerations
• Use cautiously in patients with impaired hepatic or renal function.
• Monitor for hypotension. Excessive hypotension can occur when the drug is given with a diuretic. If possible, diuretic therapy should be discontinued 2 to 3 days

(continued)

Drug therapy *(continued)*

before starting benazepril to decrease potential for excessive hypotensive response. If benazepril doesn't adequately control blood pressure, the diuretic may be restarted with care.
• Measure blood pressure when drug levels are at peak (2 to 6 hours after administration) and trough (just before a dose) to verify adequate blood pressure control.
• Assess renal and hepatic function before and periodically throughout therapy. Monitor serum potassium levels, as ordered.
• Know that other ACE inhibitors have been associated with agranulocytosis and neutropenia. Monitor complete blood count (CBC) with differential counts before therapy and periodically thereafter.

captopril
Trade name: Capoten

Adverse reactions
Common adverse reactions include agranulocytosis; angioedema of face and extremities; dry, persistent, nonproductive cough; dysgeusia; hypotension; leukopenia; maculopapular rash; pancytopenia; tachycardia; thrombocytopenia; and urticarial rash.

Special considerations
• Use cautiously in patients with impaired renal function or serious autoimmune disease (particularly systemic lupus erythematosus) or in patients who have been exposed to other drugs known to affect white blood cell (WBC) counts or immune response.
• Be aware that elderly patients may be more sensitive to the drug's hypotensive effects.
• In patients with impaired renal function or collagen vascular disease, monitor WBC and differential counts before starting treatment, every 2 weeks for the first 3 months of therapy, and periodically thereafter.

Drug therapy *(continued)*

• If pregnancy is suspected, tell patient to notify the primary care provider; the drug should be discontinued.

enalapril maleate
Trade name: Vasotec

Adverse reactions
Common adverse reactions include agranulocytosis; angioedema; dizziness; dry, persistent, tickling, nonproductive cough; dyspnea; fatigue; headache; hypotension; and neutropenia.

Special considerations
• Use cautiously in renally impaired patients.
• Monitor CBC with differential counts before and during therapy.
• Know that in patients who have diabetes, impaired renal function, or heart failure and in those who take drugs that increase serum potassium levels, hyperkalemia may develop. Monitor potassium intake and serum potassium level.
• Know that food doesn't affect absorption.
• Tell the patient to report light-headedness, signs of infection, facial swelling, difficulty breathing, or loss of taste.
• Teach the patient how to avoid orthostatic hypotension and handle it if it occurs.
• Warn the patient to seek his primary care provider's approval before taking an over-the-counter cold remedy.

fosinopril sodium
Trade name: Monopril

Adverse reactions
Common adverse reactions include cerebrovascular accident (CVA), myocardial infarction (MI), hypertensive crisis, bronchospasm, angioedema, and dry, persistent, tickling, nonproductive cough.

(continued)

Drug therapy *(continued)*

Special considerations
• Use cautiously in patients with impaired hepatic function.
• Know that diuretic therapy is usually discontinued 2 or 3 days before the start of ACE inhibitor therapy to reduce the risk of hypotension.
• Be aware that the drug's actions peak between 2 and 6 hours and last 24 hours.
• Know that other ACE inhibitors have been associated with agranulocytosis and neutropenia. Monitor CBC with differential counts, as ordered, before therapy and periodically thereafter.
• Assess hepatic function and potassium levels before and periodically throughout therapy.

---

losartan potassium
Trade name: Cozaar

Adverse reactions
Common adverse reactions include sinusitis.

Special considerations
• Use cautiously in patients with impaired renal or hepatic function.
• If pregnancy is suspected, tell patient to notify the primary care provider; the drug should be discontinued.
• Monitor the patient's blood pressure closely, especially for the first few weeks. Know that when losartan is used alone, the effect on blood pressure is notably less in black patients than in patients of other races.
• Monitor patients who also are taking diuretics for symptomatic hypotension.
• Regularly assess the patient's renal function (via serum creatinine and blood urea nitrogen [BUN] levels), as ordered.
• Be aware that patients with severe heart failure whose renal function depends on the renin-angiotensin-aldosterone system have experienced acute renal failure during ACE-inhibitor therapy. The manufacturer of losartan states that the drug

Drug therapy *(continued)*

would be expected to produce the same effect. Closely monitor the patient, especially during the first few weeks of therapy.

Alpha-adrenergic blockers

Alpha-adrenergic blockers, also known as alpha-adrenergic antagonists, act by binding to alpha receptors and preventing the release of chemicals that increase blood pressure. These drugs also reduce blood vessel tone, which diminishes peripheral vascular resistance and lowers blood pressure. As a result, alpha-adrenergic blockers are associated with postural hypotension.

Commonly used alpha-adrenergic blockers include doxazosin mesylate, labetalol hydrochloride (a combination alpha- and beta-adrenergic blocker), phentolamine mesylate, prazosin hydrochloride, and terazosin hydrochloride.

doxazosin mesylate
Trade name: Cardura

Adverse reactions
Common adverse reactions include arrhythmia, asthenia, dizziness, headache, and orthostatic hypotension.

Special considerations
• Use cautiously in patients with impaired hepatic function.
• Monitor blood pressure closely. Orthostatic effects are most likely to occur during the first 2 to 6 hours after each dose.
• Explain that orthostatic hypotension and syncope may occur, especially after the first few doses and with dosage changes. Explain how to handle hypotension and syncope if they occur.
• Advise the patient that drowsiness can occur and to avoid activities that require alertness for 24 hours after the first dose or an increase in the dose.

(continued)

Drug therapy *(continued)*

• Instruct patient to notify the primary care provider if palpitations or dizziness occurs.

labetalol hydrochloride
Trade names: Normodyne, Trandate

Adverse reactions
Common adverse reactions include bronchospasm, dizziness, orthostatic hypotension, and ventricular arrhythmia.

Special considerations
• Use cautiously in the elderly and in patients with heart failure, hepatic failure, chronic bronchitis, emphysema, preexisting peripheral vascular disease, and pheochromocytoma.
• If dizziness occurs, ask primary care provider if the patient may take a dose at bedtime or take smaller doses t.i.d. to help minimize this adverse reaction.
• Monitor blood glucose levels in diabetic patients closely because beta blockers may mask certain signs of hypoglycemia.

phentolamine mesylate
Trade name: Regitine

Adverse reactions
Common adverse reactions include arrhythmia, cerebrovascular occlusion, diarrhea, dizziness, flushing, hypotension, MI, nasal congestion, nausea, shock, vomiting, and weakness.

Special considerations
• Use cautiously in patients with gastritis or a peptic ulcer.
• Don't administer epinephrine to treat phentolamine-induced hypotension because it may cause additional fall in blood pressure ("epinephrine reversal"). Use norepinephrine instead, as ordered.

Drug therapy *(continued)*

prazosin hydrochloride

Trade name: Minipress

Adverse reactions

Common adverse reactions include dizziness, "first-dose syncope", leukopenia (transient), nausea, and palpitations.

Special considerations

- Use cautiously in patients receiving other antihypertensives.
- Know that elderly patients may be more sensitive to the drug's hypotensive effects.
- Be aware that if initial dose is greater than 1 mg, severe syncope with loss of consciousness may occur ("first-dose syncope").
- Tell the patient to notify the primary care provider if he experiences malaise or unusual adverse reactions.
- Warn patient to avoid stopping the drug abruptly; severe rebound hypertension may occur.
- Instruct the patient to avoid activities that require mental alertness until a tolerance develops to the drug's sedative effects.
- Advise patient to avoid sudden position changes to minimize orthostatic hypotension.
- Instruct patient to check with the primary care provider before taking an over-the-counter cold remedy.

terazosin hydrochloride

Trade name: Hytrin

Adverse reactions

Common adverse reactions include asthenia, dizziness, headache, nasal congestion, nausea, orthostatic hypotension, palpitations, and peripheral edema.

Special considerations

- Use cautiously in patients with renal or hepatic impairment.

(continued)

Drug therapy *(continued)*

• Monitor for hypotension and syncope during the first few days of therapy or when therapy is restarted after being interrupted for more than a few doses.
• Tell the patient to avoid tasks that require alertness for 12 hours after the first dose, an increase in the dosage, or on resumption of therapy.
• Advise patient to avoid sudden position changes to minimize orthostatic hypotension.
• Know that if terazosin is discontinued for several days, the dosage will need to be retitrated using initial dosing regimen (1 mg P.O. h.s.).
• Tell the patient to notify the primary care provider if he experiences dizziness, light-headedness, or palpitations.

Beta-adrenergic blockers

Beta-adrenergic blockers, also known as beta blockers, act by binding to $beta_1$ or $beta_2$ receptors and preventing the release of chemicals that increase blood pressure. $Beta_2$ blockers also cause peripheral vasoconstriction and bronchoconstriction. Beta blockers are commonly used in combination with diuretics. Commonly used beta blockers include acebutolol, atenolol, carteolol, metoprolol tartrate, nadolol, penbutolol sulfate, propranolol, and timolol maleate.

acebutolol

Trade name: Sectral

Adverse reactions

Common adverse reactions include arthralgia, bradycardia, bronchospasm, chest pain, constipation, cough, depression, diarrhea, dizziness, dyspepsia, dyspnea, dysuria, edema, fatigue, flatulence, headache, heart failure, hypotension, impotence, insomnia, myalgia, nausea, nocturia, rash, urinary frequency, and vomiting.

Drug therapy *(continued)*

Special considerations
• Use cautiously in patients with cardiac failure, peripheral vascular disease, bronchospastic disease, and diabetes.
• Check patient's apical pulse before giving the drug; if slower than 60 beats/minute, withhold the drug and call the primary care provider. Monitor blood pressure.
• Be aware that acebutolol may mask signs of hyperthyroidism.

atenolol
Trade name: Tenormin

Adverse reactions
Common adverse reactions include bronchospasm and heart failure.

Special considerations
• Use cautiously in patients at risk for heart failure and in those with bronchospastic disease, diabetes, hyperthyroidism, impaired renal or hepatic function, or peripheral vascular disease.
• Check patient's apical pulse before giving the drug; if slower than 60 beats/minute, withhold the drug and call the primary care provider.
• Know that the drug should be withdrawn gradually over 2 weeks to avoid serious adverse reactions.
• Instruct patient to notify the primary care provider immediately if wheezing occurs.
• Know that the drug may cause positive antinuclear antibody titers and that the drug isn't recommended for breast-feeding patients.

carteolol
Trade name: Cartrol

Adverse reactions
Common adverse reactions include asthenia, conduction disturbances, muscle cramps, and paresthesia.

(continued)

Drug therapy *(continued)*

Special considerations

• Use cautiously in patients with heart failure controlled by cardiac glycosides and diuretics because these patients may exhibit signs of heart failure with beta-blocker therapy. In addition, use cautiously in patients with hyperthyroidism or decreased pulmonary function or in breast-feeding patients.

• Know that beta blockade may inhibit glycogenolysis and mask the signs and symptoms of hypoglycemia (such as tachycardia and blood pressure changes). It may also attenuate insulin release. Monitor blood glucose levels frequently.

• Know that withdrawal of beta-blocker therapy before surgery is controversial. Some primary care providers advocate withdrawal to prevent impairment of cardiac responsiveness to reflex stimuli and decreased responsiveness to administration of catecholamines. However, the beta-blocking effects of carteolol may persist for weeks, and discontinuing the drug before surgery may be impractical. Advise the anesthesiologist that the patient is receiving a beta blocker so that isoproterenol or dobutamine is made readily available for reversal of the drug's cardiac effects.

• Be aware that patients with unrecognized coronary artery disease may exhibit signs of angina pectoris on withdrawal of the drug. Monitor closely.

• Know that a patient with diabetes may need his antidiabetic drug dosage adjusted.

• Instruct patient to notify the primary care provider if dyspnea, tachycardia, cough, or fatigue on exertion occur.

metoprolol tartrate

Trade name: Lopressor

Adverse reactions

Common adverse reactions include bradycardia, bronchospasm, dizziness, fatigue, heart failure, and hypotension.

Drug therapy *(continued)*

Special considerations
• Use cautiously in elderly patients and in those with heart failure, diabetes, or respiratory or hepatic disease.
• Always check the patient's apical pulse rate before giving the drug. If it's slower than 60 beats/minute, withhold the drug and call the primary care provider immediately.
• Monitor blood glucose levels closely in diabetic patients because the drug masks common signs of hypoglycemia.
• Know that the drug isn't recommended for breast-feeding patients.

nadolol
Trade name: Corgard

Adverse reactions
Common adverse reactions include bradycardia, heart failure, hypotension, and increased airway resistance.

Special considerations
• Use cautiously in patients with heart failure, chronic bronchitis, emphysema, or renal or hepatic impairment and in patients undergoing major surgery involving general anesthesia. Also use cautiously in patients with diabetes because beta-adrenergic blockers may mask certain signs and symptoms of hypoglycemia.
• Check patient's apical pulse before giving the drug. If slower than 60 beats/minute, withhold the drug and call the primary care provider.
• Monitor patient for signs of depression.
• Tell the patient to take the drug with meals to enhance absorption and to avoid taking the drug late in the evening to minimize insomnia.
• Know that abrupt discontinuation can exacerbate angina and precipitate an MI. The dosage should be reduced gradually over 1 to 2 weeks.
• Know that the drug isn't recommended for breast-feeding patients.
• Be aware that nadolol masks signs of shock and hyperthyroidism.

(continued)

Drug therapy *(continued)*

penbutolol sulfate
Trade name: Levatol

Adverse reactions
Common adverse reactions include bradycardia, dizziness, and heart failure.

Special considerations
• Use cautiously in patients with heart failure controlled by drug therapy and in those with a history of bronchospastic disease or who are breast-feeding. Also use cautiously in patients with diabetes because beta blockers may mask certain signs and symptoms of hypoglycemia.
• Always check the patient's apical pulse before giving the drug. If you detect extremes in pulse rates, withhold the drug and call the primary care provider immediately.
• Monitor blood pressure, electrocardiogram, and heart rate and rhythm frequently.
• Instruct patient to notify the primary care provider immediately if bradycardia, chest congestion, cough, wheezing, or dyspnea on mild exertion occur. Report all adverse reactions promptly.
• Tell the patient to check with primary care provider before taking an over-the-counter drug.

propranolol hydrochloride
Trade name: Inderal

Adverse reactions
Common adverse reactions include agranulocytosis, bradycardia, confusion, drowsiness, fatigue, heart failure, or laryngospasm.

Drug therapy *(continued)*

Special considerations

• Use cautiously in patients with renal impairment, nonallergic bronchospastic diseases, or hepatic disease and in those taking other antihypertensives. Because the drug blocks some symptoms of hypoglycemia, use with caution in patients with diabetes mellitus. Also use cautiously in patients with thyrotoxicosis because the drug may mask some signs of that disorder. Elderly patients may experience enhanced adverse reactions and may need dosage adjustment.

• Always check the patient's apical pulse before giving the drug. If you detect extremes in pulse rates, withhold the drug and call the patient's primary care provider immediately.

• Give consistently with meals. Food may increase absorption of propranolol.

• Be aware that the drug masks common signs of shock.

• Tell the patient not to stop taking the drug abruptly; rebound hypertension, MI, or palpitations may occur.

• Advise the patient to avoid tasks requiring mental alertness until reaction to the drug is known.

• Tell patient to check with primary care provider before taking an over-the-counter drug.

timolol maleate

Trade name: Blocadren

Adverse reactions

Common adverse reactions include arrhythmia, bronchospasm, CVA, cardiac arrest, and heart failure.

Special considerations

• Use cautiously in patients with heart failure; hepatic, renal, or respiratory disease; diabetes; and hyperthyroidism.

• Avoid use in breast-feeding patients.

(continued)

Drug therapy *(continued)*

• Check the patient's apical pulse rate before giving the drug. If you detect extremes in pulse rates, withhold the drug and call the primary care provider.
• Monitor blood glucose levels in diabetic patients; the drug can mask signs and symptoms of hypoglycemia.

Calcium channel blockers

Calcium channel blockers inhibit the flow of calcium into cardiac and vascular cells. With less calcium in the cells, blood vessels dilate and cardiac output decreases, which lowers blood pressure. Commonly used calcium channel blockers include amlodipine besylate, isradipine, nicardipine hydrochloride, and verapamil hydrochloride.

amlodipine besylate
Trade name: Norvasc

Adverse reactions
Common adverse reactions include edema, headache, and light-headedness.

Special considerations
• Use cautiously in patients receiving other peripheral vasodilators, especially those with aortic stenosis, heart failure, or severe hepatic disease.
• Monitor the patient carefully. Some patients, especially those with severe obstructive coronary artery disease, have developed increased frequency, duration, or severity of angina or even an acute MI after initiation of calcium channel blocker therapy or at time of dosage increase.
• Monitor blood pressure frequently during initiation of therapy. Because the drug-induced vasodilation has a gradual onset, acute hypotension is rare.
• Notify the primary care provider if signs of heart failure occur, such as swelling of hands and feet or shortness of breath.

Drug therapy *(continued)*

isradipine
Trade name: DynaCirc

Adverse reactions
Common adverse reactions include headache.

Special considerations
• Use cautiously in patients with heart failure, especially if combined with a beta blocker, and in patients with renal or hepatic impairment.
• Monitor the patient for adverse reactions. Like other calcium channel blockers, isradipine is known to cause symptomatic hypotension. Most adverse reactions are mild and transient and related to vasodilation (dizziness, edema, flushing, palpitations, and tachycardia).
• Before surgery, inform the anesthesiologist that the patient is taking a calcium channel blocker.

nicardipine hydrochloride
Trade name: Cardene

Adverse reactions
Common adverse reactions include asthenia, dizziness, flushing, headache, light-headedness, palpitations, or paresthesia.

Special considerations
• Use cautiously in patients with hypotension, heart failure, impaired hepatic or renal function, cardiac conduction disturbance, or advanced aortic stenosis.
• Measure blood pressure frequently during initial therapy. Maximum blood pressure response occurs about 1 hour after dosing with the immediate-release form and 2 to 4 hours with the sustained-release form. Check for potential orthostatic

(continued)

Drug therapy *(continued)*

hypotension. Because large swings in blood pressure may occur based on blood level of the drug, assess adequacy of antihypertensive effect 8 hours after dosing.
• Avoid use in breast-feeding patients.

---

verapamil hydrochloride
Trade names: Calan SR, Isoptin SR

Adverse reactions
Common adverse reactions include constipation, heart failure, transient hypotension, ventricular asystole, and ventricular fibrillation.

Special considerations
• Use cautiously in elderly patients, in patients with increased intracranial pressure, and in patients with hepatic or renal disease.
• Although the drug should be taken with food, be aware that taking extended-release tablets with food may decrease rate and extent of absorption but allows smaller fluctuations of peak and trough blood levels.
• Patients who have severely compromised cardiac function or who take carbamazepine, digoxin, or a beta blocker should receive a lower dose of verapamil. Monitor these patients closely.
• Teach the patient to rise slowly to reduce orthostatic hypotension.
• Monitor blood pressure at the start of therapy and during dosage adjustments.
• Notify the primary care provider if signs of heart failure, such as swelling of hands and feet or shortness of breath, occur.

Centrally acting antiadrenergics

Centrally acting antiadrenergics decrease the release of adrenergic hormones from the brain, thus reducing peripheral vascular resistance and blood pressure without diminishing blood flow to organs. These drugs are most helpful for patients with

Drug therapy *(continued)*

decreased renal function. Commonly used centrally acting antiadrenergics include clonidine hydrochloride, guanabenz acetate, and guanfacine hydrochloride.

---

clonidine hydrochloride

Trade name: Catapres

Adverse reactions

Common adverse reactions include constipation, dermatitis (with transdermal patch), dizziness, drowsiness, dry mouth, pruritus, rash, sedation, and severe rebound hypertension.

Special considerations

- Use cautiously in patients with severe coronary insufficiency, recent MI, cerebrovascular disease, chronic renal failure, or impaired liver function.
- Know that clonidine may be given to rapidly lower blood pressure in some hypertensive emergencies.
- Antihypertensive effects of transdermal clonidine may take 2 to 3 days to become apparent. Oral antihypertensive therapy may have to be continued in the interim.
- Remove transdermal patch before defibrillation to prevent arcing.
- When stopping therapy in patients receiving both clonidine and a beta blocker, gradually withdraw the beta blocker first to minimize adverse reactions, as ordered, and then taper the dosage to prevent rebound effect.
- Notify the primary care provider if the patient gains more than 4 lb in one week.
- Instruct patient to avoid tasks that require alertness until tolerance to the drug's sedative effects develops.
- Advise the patient to rise slowly to reduce orthostatic hypotension.
- Instruct the patient to check with the primary care provider before taking an over-the-counter cold remedy.
- Be aware that discontinuation in preparation for surgery isn't recommended, nor is use in breast-feeding patients.

(continued)

Drug therapy *(continued)*

guanabenz acetate
Trade name: Wytensin

Adverse reactions
Common adverse reactions include dizziness, drowsiness, dry mouth, rebound hypertension, sedation, and weakness.

Special considerations
• Use cautiously in patients with severe coronary insufficiency, a recent MI, cerebrovascular disease, or severe hepatic or renal failure. Also use cautiously in elderly patients.
• Store the drug in a light-resistant container.
• Avoid stopping the drug abruptly; severe rebound hypertension may occur.
• Advise the patient to take the last dose at bedtime to minimize daytime drowsiness and ensure overnight control of the blood pressure.
• Instruct the patient to avoid tasks that require alertness until tolerance to the drug's sedative effects develops.
• Instruct the patient to check with the primary care provider before taking an over-the-counter cold remedy.

guanfacine hydrochloride
Trade name: Tenex

Adverse reactions
Common adverse reactions include constipation, dizziness, dry mouth, and somnolence.

Special considerations
• Use cautiously in patients with severe coronary insufficiency, a recent MI, cerebrovascular disease, or chronic renal or hepatic insufficiency.

Drug therapy *(continued)*

• Be aware that the incidence and severity of adverse reactions increase with higher dosage and that incidence of these reactions decreases with continued use.
• Advise the patient to take the last dose at bedtime to minimize daytime drowsiness and ensure overnight control of blood pressure.
• Instruct the patient to avoid tasks that require alertness until tolerance to the drug's sedative effects develops.
• Advise the patient to avoid alcohol and other CNS depressants, which may increase drowsiness.
• Instruct the patient to notify the primary care provider before taking an over-the-counter cold remedy.

Diuretics

Sodium and water levels can affect blood volume and influence blood pressure. Diuretics can reduce blood pressure by reducing sodium and water retention in the body. Thiazide-based diuretics, such as chlorothiazide, chlorthalidone, and hydrochlorothiazide, are considered first-line drugs for hypertension. Loop diuretics, such as bumetanide, ethacrynate sodium, and furosemide, inhibit sodium reabsorption in the loop of Henle. Potassium-sparing diuretics, such as amiloride hydrochloride and spironolactone, cause the kidneys to excrete water and sodium without depleting potassium.

amiloride hydrochloride
Trade name: Midamor

Adverse reactions
Common adverse reactions include abdominal pain, anorexia, aplastic anemia, appetite changes, constipation, diarrhea, dizziness, dyspnea, encephalopathy, fatigue, headache, hyperkalemia, hyponatremia, impotence, muscle cramps, nausea, neutropenia, orthostatic hypotension, vomiting, and weakness.

(continued)

Drug therapy (continued)

Special considerations
• Use cautiously in patients with diabetes mellitus, cardiopulmonary disease, and severe existing renal or hepatic insufficiency and in elderly or debilitated patients.
• To prevent nausea, administer the drug with meals.
• If the drug isn't taken concurrently with a potassium-wasting drug, monitor potassium level because of increased risk of hyperkalemia. Alert the primary care provider immediately if potassium level exceeds 6.5 mEq/L, and expect the drug to be discontinued.

bumetanide
Trade name: Bumex

Adverse reactions
Common adverse reactions include renal failure, thrombocytopenia, and weakness.

Special considerations
• Use cautiously in the elderly and in patients with depressed renal or hepatic function.
• To prevent nocturia, give in the morning. If second dose is necessary, give in early afternoon.
• Be aware that the safest and most effective dosage schedule for controlling edema is intermittent dosage given on alternate days or for 3 to 4 days with 1 to 2 days of rest.
• Monitor fluid intake and output, weight, and serum electrolyte, BUN, creatinine, and carbon dioxide levels frequently.
• Watch for evidence of hypokalemia, such as muscle weakness and cramps. Instruct the patient to report these symptoms.
• Consult the primary care provider and dietitian about a high-potassium diet. Foods rich in potassium include citrus fruits, tomatoes, bananas, dates, and apricots.
• Monitor blood glucose levels in diabetic patients.

Drug therapy *(continued)*

- Monitor blood uric acid levels, especially in patients with history of gout.
- Monitor blood pressure and pulse rate during rapid diuresis. Bumetanide can lead to profound water and electrolyte depletion.
- If oliguria or azotemia develops or increases, know that the primary care provider may stop the drug.
- Keep in mind that bumetanide can be safely used in patients allergic to furosemide.

chlorthalidone
Trade name: Hygroton

Adverse reactions
Common adverse reactions include agranulocytosis, aplastic anemia, dizziness, dyspepsia, electrolyte imbalances, photosensitivity, and restlessness.

Special considerations
- Use cautiously in elderly patients and in those with renal impairment.
- Instruct the patient in how to handle orthostatic hypotension.
- As ordered, discontinue the drug prior to parathyroid function tests.

chlorothiazide
Trade name: Diuril

Adverse reactions
Common adverse reactions include agranulocytosis, anaphylactic reaction, aplastic anemia, dry mouth, hyperglycemia, hypokalemia, and photosensitivity.

Special considerations
- Use cautiously in patients with impaired renal function.
- Avoid infiltration or extravasation; the drug is extremely irritating to tissues. If infiltration or extravasation occurs, discontinue the infusion and apply ice.

(continued)

Drug therapy *(continued)*

• Notify the primary care provider if the patient gains more than 2 lb in 3 days, experiences prolonged vomiting or diarrhea, or exhibits signs and symptoms of hypokalemia, hypercalcemia, or hyperglycemia.
• Advise the patient to take the drug in the morning with food to avoid GI upset.
• Consult the primary care provider and dietitian about a high-potassium diet. Foods rich in potassium include citrus fruits, tomatoes, bananas, apricots, and dates.

---

ethacrynate sodium
Trade name: Sodium Edecrin

Adverse reactions
Common adverse reactions include agranulocytosis, neutropenia, and thrombocytopenia.

Special considerations
• Use cautiously in patients with electrolyte abnormalities, diabetes, or renal or hepatic impairment.
• Give oral doses in the morning to prevent nocturia.
• Do not give S.C. or I.M. because of local pain and irritation.
• Watch for signs of hypokalemia, such as muscle weakness and cramps.
• Consult the primary care provider and dietitian about providing a high-potassium diet. Foods rich in potassium include citrus fruits, tomatoes, bananas, dates, and apricots. Know that potassium chloride and sodium supplements may be needed.
• Monitor blood uric acid levels, especially in patients with a history of gout.
• Be aware that severe diarrhea will necessitate discontinuing the drug. Know that the patient should not receive the drug again after diarrhea has resolved.
• Know that rapid injection may cause transient deafness and hypotension.
• Periodically assess hearing function in a patient receiving high doses. The drug may also increase the risk of ototoxicity from other drugs.

Drug therapy *(continued)*

furosemide
Trade name: Lasix

Adverse reactions
Common adverse reactions include agranulocytosis, aplastic anemia, and thrombocytopenia.

Special considerations
• Use cautiously in patients with renal or hepatic impairment. Know that furosemide should be used during pregnancy only if potential benefits clearly outweigh possible risks to fetus.
• To prevent nocturia, give P.O. and I.V. preparations in the morning. Give second doses in early afternoon.
• Monitor weight, blood pressure, and pulse rate routinely with long-term use and during rapid diuresis. Furosemide can lead to profound water and electrolyte depletion.
• Monitor blood uric acid level, especially in patients with a history of gout.
• Notify the primary care provider if oliguria or azotemia develops or increases; it may require stopping the drug.
• Watch for signs of hypokalemia, such as muscle weakness and cramps.
• Consult the primary care provider and dietitian about a high-potassium diet. Foods rich in potassium include citrus fruits, tomatoes, bananas, and dates.
• Know that oral furosemide may not be well absorbed in a patient with severe heart failure. The drug may need to be given I.V. even if the patient is taking other oral medications.
• Be aware that discolored tablets or injectable solution should not be used.

(continued)

Drug therapy *(continued)*

hydrochlorothiazide
Trade names: Esidrix, HydroDIURIL, Oretic

Adverse reactions
Common adverse reactions include agranulocytosis, anaphylactic reaction, aplastic anemia, renal failure, and thrombocytopenia.

Special considerations
• Use cautiously in children and in patients with severe renal disease, impaired hepatic function, diabetes, or progressive hepatic disease.
• To prevent nocturia, give in the morning or early afternoon.
• Monitor fluid intake and output, weight, blood pressure, and serum electrolyte levels.
• Watch for signs of hypokalemia, such as muscle weakness and cramps. The drug may be used with potassium sparing diuretic to prevent potassium loss.
• Consult the primary care provider and dietitian about a high-potassium diet. Foods rich in potassium include citrus fruits, tomatoes, bananas, apricots, and dates.
• Monitor serum creatinine and BUN levels regularly. Cumulative effects of the drug may occur with impaired renal function.
• Monitor blood uric acid levels, especially in patients with history of gout.
• Monitor blood glucose levels, especially in diabetic patients.
• Monitor elderly patients, who are especially susceptible to excessive diuresis.
• As ordered, discontinue thiazides and thiazide-like diuretics before parathyroid function tests.
• In patients with hypertension, know that therapeutic response may be delayed several weeks.
• Tell the patient to report changes in hearing, signs of hypovolemia or electrolyte imbalances (confusion, dizziness, headache, muscle cramps, and paresthesia).

Drug therapy *(continued)*

- Teach the patient how to handle orthostatic hypotension.
- Instruct the patient to use a sunscreen to avoid skin damage due to photosensitivity.
- Instruct the patient to check with the primary care provider before taking an over-the-counter cold remedy.

---

spironolactone

Trade name: Aldactone

Adverse reactions

Common adverse reactions include agranulocytosis and hyperkalemia.

Special considerations

- Use cautiously in patients with fluid or electrolyte imbalances, impaired renal function, and hepatic disease.
- Spironolactone or its metabolites may cross the placental barrier. Use with extreme caution in pregnancy.
- To enhance absorption, give the drug with meals.
- Inform the laboratory that the patient is taking spironolactone, because it may interfere with certain laboratory tests that measure digoxin level.
- Although the drug is less potent than thiazide and loop diuretics, it's useful as an adjunct to other diuretic therapy. The diuretic effect is delayed 2 to 3 days when used alone.
- Keep in mind that maximum antihypertensive response may be delayed for up to 2 weeks.
- Watch for signs and symptoms of hyperchloremic metabolic acidosis in patients with hepatic cirrhosis.
- Know that tumor development has been reported in some patients taking spironolactone.

(continued)

Drug therapy *(continued)*

Vasodilators

Vasodilators reduce blood pressure by relaxing the smooth-muscle lining of blood vessels. Certain vasodilators such as diazoxide are most effective when used in combination with a beta blocker and a diuretic. Others vasodilators such as nitroprusside sodium are usually reserved for hypertensive emergencies. Commonly used vasodilators include diazoxide, hydralazine hydrochloride, minoxidil, and nitroprusside sodium.

---

diazoxide

Trade name: Hyperstat IV

Adverse reactions

Common adverse reactions include abdominal discomfort, angina, arrhythmia, cerebral ischemia, hyperglycemia, hyperosmotic hyperglycemic nonketotic syndrome, hyperuricemia, ketoacidosis, MI, nausea, orthostatic hypotension, paralysis, seizures, shock, sodium and water retention, thrombocytopenia, and vomiting.

Special considerations

• Use cautiously in patients with impaired cerebral or cardiac function or uremia.
• Check the patient's standing blood pressure before discontinuing close monitoring for hypotension.
• Monitor the patient's fluid intake and output carefully. If fluid or sodium retention develops, the patient's primary care provider may order diuretics.
• Weigh the patient daily and notify the primary care provider of weight increase of more than 4 lb per week.
• Don't use solution if it's discolored or if particles are visible.
• Know that diazoxide may alter requirements for insulin, diet, or oral antidiabetic drugs in patients with previously controlled diabetes. Monitor blood glucose level

Drug therapy *(continued)*

daily; watch for signs of severe hyperglycemia or hyperosmolar hyperglycemic nonketotic syndrome. Insulin may be needed.
• Check uric acid levels frequently and report abnormalities to the primary care provider.
• Teach the patient how to handle orthostatic hypotension.

hydralazine hydrochloride
Trade name: Apresoline

Adverse reactions
Common adverse reactions include agranulocytosis, angina, anorexia, diarrhea, headache, lupuslike syndrome (especially with high doses), nausea, palpitations, shock, tachycardia, and vomiting.

Special considerations
• Use cautiously in patients with suspected cardiac disease, CVA, or severe renal impairment and in those taking other antihypertensives.
• Monitor the patient's blood pressure, pulse rate, and body weight frequently. Some primary care providers combine hydralazine therapy with diuretics and beta blockers to decrease sodium retention and tachycardia and prevent angina attacks.
• Be aware that headache and palpitations may occur 2 to 4 hours after the first oral dose but should subside spontaneously.
• Monitor CBC, lupus erythematosus cell preparation, and antinuclear antibody titer determination before therapy and periodically during long-term therapy, as ordered.
• Watch the patient closely for signs of lupuslike syndrome (sore throat, fever, muscle and joint aches, and rash). Notify the primary care provider immediately if these develop.
• Teach the patient how to handle orthostatic hypotension.
• Know that some preparations contain tartrazine, which may cause allergic reaction in patients sensitive to aspirin.

(continued)

Drug therapy *(continued)*

• Notify the primary care provider for weight gain greater than 5 lb per week.
• Advise patient to check with the primary care provider before taking an over-the-counter cold remedy.

minoxidil
Trade name: Loniten

Adverse reactions
Common adverse reactions include breast tenderness, edema, heart failure, hypertrichosis (elongation, thickening, and enhanced pigmentation of fine body hair), nausea, pericardial effusion and tamponade, Stevens-Johnson syndrome, tachycardia, and weight gain.

Special considerations
• Use cautiously in patients with impaired renal function and after an acute MI.
• Closely monitor blood pressure and pulse at beginning of therapy.
• Monitor for heart failure, pericardial effusion, and cardiac tamponade. Have emergency drugs available to treat hypotension.
• Notify the primary care provider of heart rate more than 20 beats per minute over normal, rapid weight gain, shortness of breath, dizziness, light-headedness, or syncope.
• Advise the patient to check with the primary care provider before taking an over-the-counter cold remedy.
• Be sure to administer dose after dialysis.

nitroprusside sodium
Trade name: Nitropress

Adverse reactions
Common adverse reactions include abdominal pain, cyanide toxicity, diaphoresis, dizziness, headache, increased intracranial pressure (ICP), methemoglobinemia, muscle twitching, nausea, rash, and thiocyanate toxicity.

Drug therapy *(continued)*

Special considerations

• Use with extreme caution in patients with increased ICP. Use cautiously in patients with hypothyroidism, hepatic or renal disease, hyponatremia, or low vitamin B_{12} concentration.
• Obtain baseline vital signs before giving the drug, and find out what parameters the patient's primary care provider wants to achieve.
• Keep the patient in the supine position when initiating or titrating the drug.
• Check the patient's blood pressure every 15 minutes throughout an infusion of nitroprusside sodium.
• Don't use bacteriostatic water for injection or normal saline solution to prepare the solution; use dextrose 5% in water.
• Wrap I.V. solution container (but not the tubing) in aluminum foil; the solution is light-sensitive. Discard solutions after 24 hours.

safely begin taking lower drug dosages. In such cases, the dosage is gradually reduced and the patient monitored regularly for adverse reactions. (See *Follow-up guidelines, page 94.*)

Surgical treatment

Surgical treatment for hypertension is used when the patient suffers from pheochromocytoma — a tumor usually found in the medulla of the adrenal gland. The tumor can produce large amounts of epinephrine and norepinephrine, both of which raise blood pressure, sometimes severely. The tumors are equally as common in men and women and usually occur between ages 30 and 60.

Battling illness

Follow-up guidelines

Blood pressure measurements reflect the average of three or more readings, taken over 1 to 2 weeks. The diagram below provides current follow-up guidelines for patients ages 18 and older who have hypertension and who don't have other conditions or signs of organ damage from hypertension. Patients who have signs of organ damage or other health conditions need more aggressive management. A blood pressure of 210 mm Hg or higher systolic or 120 mm Hg or higher diastolic requires emergency treatment.

Diastolic blood pressure (mm Hg)	Systolic blood pressure (mm Hg)				
	Below 130	130 to 139	140 to 159	160 to 179	180 to 209
Below 85	Recheck within 2 years				
85 to 89	Recheck within 1 year				
90 to 99	Recheck within 2 months				
100 to 109	Recheck within 1 month; refer for care				
110 to 119	Recheck within 24 hours; refer for care				

Removing the tumor

Surgical removal of the tumor is the treatment of choice. Because high levels of epinephrine can make surgery danger-

Battling illness

Ethnic differences in drug response

Antihypertensive and other cardiac agents display differences in their effectiveness among Black, White, and Asian patients. For example, Black patients respond better to thiazide diuretics, whereas White patients respond better to angiotensin-converting enzyme inhibitors such as captopril. Asian patients are twice as responsive to propranolol's effects on blood pressure and heart rate as White patients.

Plasma renin activity may account for this difference in drug response because it varies by ethnic group. For example, White patients usually have a higher rate of plasma renin activity than Black patients.

ous, surgery can't be performed until the high levels of epinephrine and norepinephrine are controlled. Phenoxybenzamine and propranolol are the drugs of choice to lower and control these levels. (See *Ethnic differences in drug response.*)

Quick quiz

1. The preferred drugs for the initial treatment of hypertension include:
- A. adrenergic blockers and calcium channel blockers.
- B. diuretics and beta blockers.
- C. vasodilators and angiotensin II blockers.

Answer: B. Diuretics and beta blockers are usually the first medications prescribed for patients with hypertension.

2. Calcium channel blockers work by:
- A. inhibiting the release of norepinephrine and calcium.
- B. inhibiting the flow of calcium into cardiac and vascular cells.
- C. promoting sodium and calcium excretion through the loop of Henle.

Answer: B. Calcium channel blockers inhibit the flow of calcium into cardiac and vascular cells.

3. Pheochromocytoma, a tumor of the adrenal gland, can produce large amounts of:

    A. insulin.

    B. sodium and potassium.

    C. norepinephrine and epinephrine.

Answer: C. Pheochromocytomas can produce large amounts of norepinephrine and epinephrine, which can raise blood pressure.

4. Adrenergic blockers are usually reserved for patients:

    A. with pheochromocytoma.

    B. who respond favorably to mild diuretics.

    C. who don't respond to other medications.

Answer: C. Adrenergic blockers are usually reserved for patients who don't respond to other antihypertensives.

5. The drugs of choice to control high levels of epinephrine and norepinephrine in pheochromocytoma include:

    A. insulin and dobutamine.

    B. phenoxybenzamine and propranolol.

    C. propranolol and labetalol.

Answer: B. Phenoxybenzamine and propranolol are the drugs of choice to lower and control levels of epinephrine and norepinephrine in patients with pheochromocytoma.

Scoring

☆☆☆ If you answered all five questions correctly, super! You've followed the four-step process to success!

☆☆ If you answered four questions correctly, good job! Keep your studying at current dosage levels.

☆ If you answered three or fewer questions correctly, don't worry. Additional review is the treatment of choice for this chapter.

5

Complications

> ### Key facts
> ◆ Sustained, untreated hypertension can lead to organ damage affecting the heart, brain, kidneys, and eyes.
> ◆ Hypertensive crisis and malignant hypertension are emergency complications demanding immediate treatment.
> ◆ Pregnancy-related hypertension can produce serious complications such as preeclampsia.

Cardiac complications

A number of cardiac-related complications of hypertension can occur, including heart failure, coronary artery disease (CAD), and dissecting aortic aneurysm.

Heart failure

Heart failure results from the inability of the heart to pump a sufficient volume of blood to meet the meta-

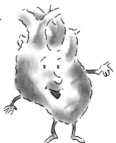

bolic needs of the body. Hypertension increases the heart's workload, raising the risk of heart failure.

Signs and symptoms of heart failure depend on whether the patient suffers right- or left-sided heart failure.

Heart failure on the right

Right-sided heart failure stems from the inability of the right ventricle to empty completely. Unable to pump out all its blood with each contraction, blood begins to pool in the right ventricle and, eventually, back up into the superior and inferior venae cavae.

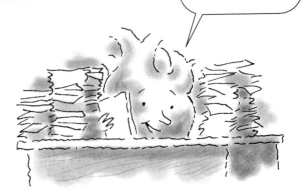

Hypertension increases my workload, making it harder for me to pump all that blood.

Right-sided heart failure usually results in a buildup of fluid throughout the body. Look for the following signs:
- jugular vein distention
- leg and ankle edema
- liver enlargement.

Heart failure on the left

Left-sided failure stems from the inability of the left ventricle to empty completely. As a result, blood pools in the ventricle and backs up into the pulmonary circulation.

Left-sided heart failure usually results in a buildup of fluid in the lungs. Look for the following signs and symptoms:
- dyspnea
- fatigue
- orthopnea
- paroxysmal nocturnal dyspnea.

> When the heart fails on the left side, fluid builds up in poor ol' me.

Treat with rest and drugs

If the patient has severe heart failure, he should limit activity, as necessary, for several days. He'll also take such drugs as diuretics and vasodilators to reduce his blood pressure, and he may take a cardiac glycoside, such as digoxin, to improve myocardial contraction.

Because excess weight increases stress on the heart, monitor the patient's weight daily, and report a gain of 2 lb (0.9 kg) or more a week.

CAD

Damage to the coronary arteries as a result of sustained hypertension can cause fatty deposits, or plaques, to form inside arteries. These plaques can build up and, if they grow large enough to block an artery, can cause acute myocardial infarction (MI).

CAD's big symptom: Chest pain

The main symptom of CAD is angina. Angina typically produces pain or a tightness in the chest, left shoulder or arm, back, jaw, or right arm. The pain of stable angina usually occurs with exertion. The pain of unstable angina usually occurs with little exertion or at rest.

Treat with drugs

Stable and unstable angina are typically treated with drug therapy. Nitrates reduce chest pain, while beta blockers may

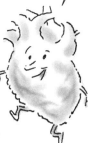

If my angina is stable, I cause pain with exertion.

be used to lower blood pressure. Calcium channel blockers can also alleviate symptoms by reducing the patient's heart rate. In severe cases, coronary artery bypass surgery or angioplasty may be used to restore blood flow to the heart.

Dissecting aortic aneurysm

As a result of stretching from long-term, severe hypertension, medial fibers in the aorta may rupture, resulting in dissecting aortic aneurysm. A dissected aorta may cause sudden, severe chest pain.

Pain may also occur between the scapulas, and you may detect decreased or absent pulses in the arms or legs. The patient may also have a heart murmur or signs of cardiac tamponade.

Treat with surgery

The patient with a dissecting aortic aneurysm needs surgery to replace the dissected aorta with a synthetic graft. Drugs can also be used to control the patient's heart rate and blood pressure.

If my angina is unstable, I cause pain at rest.

Central nervous system complications

Hypertension can cause several central nervous system complications, including cerebrovascular accident (CVA), hypertensive encephalopathy, and hypertensive retinopathy.

CVA

Over time, hypertension can lead to a rupture or blockage of a cerebral blood vessel. Depending on its location, this rupture or blockage can result in cerebral ischemia or death of cerebral tissue distal to the problem area.

Slurred speech may signal

Signs and symptoms of CVA can be numerous and generally depend on which part of the brain has suffered damage. Common signs and symptoms include:
- confusion
- difficulty swallowing
- headache
- hemiplegia
- slurred speech or aphasia.

Treat with drugs and rehab

Treatment for a CVA may include diuretics to reduce hypertension and anticoagulants if the CVA resulted from an embolism. Maintain a patent airway for the patient and provide him with nutrition I.V. or through a nasogastric tube. Rehabilitation for a CVA may include physical and speech therapy.

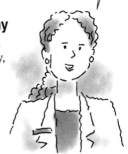

Signs and symptoms of a CVA vary depending on the area affected.

Hypertensive encephalopathy

Severe, prolonged hypertension can lead to hypertensive encephalopathy, or swelling of the brain. The condition can cause drowsiness or even coma. The patient may also experience seizures or retinopathy with papilledema.

Drop the pressure fast

Hypertensive encephalopathy requires prompt lowering of arterial blood pressure to prevent life-threatening symptoms. Rapid-acting antihypertensive drugs are commonly used to quickly relieve blood pressure.

Hypertensive retinopathy

The main eye-related complication of severe hypertension is hypertensive retinopathy. In this disorder, damage to the blood vessels of the retina of the eye can cause blood to leak into the retina and the optic nerve to swell. In severe cases, the patient may experience blurred vision or even blindness.

Retinal damage from hypertension can cause blurred vision or even blindness.

I spy arterial narrowing

Hypertensive retinopathy may be detected through funduscopic examination of the eye. The disorder is graded on a scale of I to IV:
• grade I — arterial narrowing or spasm
• grade II — arteriovenous nicking
• grade III — hemorrhages and exudates
• grade IV — papilledema.
The condition is treated with antihypertensive drugs.

Renal complications

Severe hypertension can cause thickening of renal arterioles. As the arterioles thicken, the kidneys lose their ability to filter waste products from the blood, which ultimately leads to renal failure.

Early signs and symptoms

Signs and symptoms of renal failure may develop slowly. In its early stages, renal failure may cause:
- anorexia
- edema
- nausea
- proteinuria
- weakness.

Latecomers

If left untreated, end-stage failure can develop, causing:
- generalized itching
- headache
- severe lethargy
- stomatitis
- vomiting.

Treating renal failure

Treatment for early renal failure includes placing the patient on a low-protein diet, maintaining his electrolyte and fluid balance, and using antihypertensive drugs to lower the blood pressure. End-stage

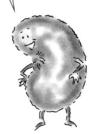

Hypertension makes my arterioles thick. I can't do my job right with thick arterioles.

renal failure may require dialysis or kidney transplantation.

Emergency complications

On occasion, hypertension can lead to conditions requiring emergency evaluation and treatment. The most critical of those conditions include malignant hypertension and hypertensive crisis.

Malignant hypertension

Malignant hypertension is a severe, fulminant form of hypertension that can arise from either essential or secondary hypertension. Malignant hypertension usually involves a diastolic pressure near 130 mm Hg or higher.

Watch out!

When blood pressure climbs that high, the patient may experience:
- papilledema
- retinal hemorrhage and exudates
- severe headache
- vomiting
- transient paralysis
- stupor

- seizures
- coma.

Take the I.V. train

To quickly reduce blood pressure, administer drugs I.V. When delivered I.V., diazoxide (Hyperstat IV) can reduce blood pressure in 1 to 3 minutes. Nitroprusside (Nitropress) may also be given I.V. Hydralazine (Apresoline) or methyldopa (Aldomet) can help the patient maintain long-term control of malignant hypertension.

Hypertensive crisis

In hypertensive crisis, arterial blood pressure rises rapidly and severely, threatening the patient's life. If left untreated, this condition can quickly compromise the patient's cerebral, cardiovascular, and renal function.

How much of an emergency?

Hypertensive crisis can be divided into two categories, hypertensive emergency and hypertensive urgency.

Hypertensive emergency is immediately life-threatening. Situations in which

controlling hypertension is considered
an emergency include hypertensive encephalopathy, acute aortic dissection,
pulmonary edema, pheochromocytoma
crisis, monoamine oxidase inhibitor and
tyramine interaction, intracranial hemorrhage, and eclampsia. I.V. antihypertensives must be used to lower blood pressure in a period of a few minutes to 1
hour. (See *Risks of emergency antihyper-*
tensives, page 112.)

Hypertensive urgency is less immediately life-threatening. Situations in
which controlling hypertension
would be considered urgent include CAD, kidney transplantation, and accelerated, malignant
hypertension. Patients in the post-
operative period and in situations
requiring emergency surgery also
fall into this category. Oral antihypertensives or slower-acting parenteral
drugs can be used to lower pressure
within 24 hours.

> Given
> through my
> line,
> diazoxide
> can reduce
> blood
> pressure in
> under 3
> minutes.

What to watch for

If a patient with extremely high blood
pressure develops a severe headache,

blurred vision, or nausea and vomiting, he may be having a hypertensive crisis. Other signs and symptoms include:

- azotemia
- chest pain
- dyspnea
- leg and arm numbness or tingling
- oliguria
- progressive impairment of consciousness
- retinal hemorrhagic exudates and papilledema.

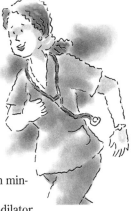

In a hypertensive emergency, you may have only a few minutes to react.

Treating the emergency

Hypertensive emergency can be treated with rapid-acting antihypertensives such as:

- nitroprusside (Nitropress), a vasodilator that acts directly on smooth muscle of arterioles within minutes
- diazoxide (Hyperstat IV), a vasodilator that acts within 1 minute to dilate arteriolar smooth muscle
- hydralazine (Apresoline), a vasodilator that acts directly on arteriolar smooth muscle within 20 minutes when given I.V. or within 30 minutes when given I.M.

Before you give that drug

Risks of emergency antihypertensives

Emergency antihypertensives can pose their own risks. To ensure the patient's safety, be aware of proper infusion rates, especially with diazoxide, esmolol, or nitroprusside.

Diazoxide

To reduce the danger of a stroke or a myocardial infarction when using diazoxide, use serial low-dose I.V. injections. These injections reduce blood pressure more gradually than a single large bolus dose and pose less danger of cardiovascular complications.

Esmolol

Assess baseline breath sounds during your initial assessment and then periodically during the infusion to detect signs and symptoms of heart failure from esmolol. Assess for wheezing; esmolol can also cause bronchospasm. In addition, monitor the patient's heart rate and blood pressure; this drug may cause bradycardia.

Nitroprusside

Nitroprusside infusion carries a risk of lethal cyanide toxicity, life-threatening hypotension, and thiocyanate toxicity. Avoid these effects by:

• administering the drug for short durations and at slow infusion rates (under 2 mcg/kg/minute)

• starting the infusion at 0.3 mcg/kg/minute and titrating upward until the desired effect is achieved or the maximum recommended dose is reached

• infusing for a maximum of 10 minutes when the maximum rate of 10 mcg/kg/minute is being given.

• labetalol (Normodyne, Trandate), an alpha- and beta-adrenergic blocker that acts within 5 minutes to reduce blood pressure.

Treating the urgency

Hypertensive urgency is treated with antihypertensives such as:

• nifedipine (Adalat, Procardia), a calcium channel blocker that begins acting in about 20 minutes to lower blood pressure

• clonidine (Catapres), a centrally acting antihypertensive that begins acting in under 1 hour

• captopril (Capoten), an angiotensin-converting enzyme (ACE) inhibitor that begins acting within 1 hour and may act as quickly as 15 minutes

• enalaprilat (Vasotec I.V.), a potent ACE inhibitor that begins to act 5 to 15 minutes after being given I.V.

This captopril we're giving you will help control your blood pressure. We should see results within about an hour.

Hypertension and pregnancy

Hypertension can produce serious consequences for a pregnant patient and her fetus. Pregnancy normally prompts changes in blood pressure, but in some cases, these changes can reach hypertensive levels.

Blood pressure changes

In normal pregnancy, the number of red blood cells and other plasma components increases and the renin-angiotensin-aldosterone system accelerates. These effects result in an expansion of blood volume by 30% to 50%, which increases stroke volume, heart rate, and cardiac output. Arterioles dilate and peripheral vascular resistance drops.

As a result, blood pressure generally drops slightly in the first trimester, and continues to drop through the second trimester. Blood pressure rises again during the third trimester.

Pressure regulators, don't fail me now

When the body's normal blood pressure regulation system fails during pregnancy, the patient may develop:

• chronic hypertension, noted by a blood pressure of 140/90 mm Hg before the 20th week of gestation and possibly persisting after delivery

• late or transient hypertension, noted by a blood pressure that increases during labor or early postpartum and returns to normal within 10 days after delivery

• pregnancy-induced hypertension (PIH), which occurs after the 20th week of gestation. PIH constitutes the most serious blood pressure–related pregnancy disorder.

Watch for transient hypertension during labor. This form of hypertension generally returns to normal within 10 days.

Preeclampsia

PIH can occur as preeclampsia or, in its most severe form, eclampsia. In preeclampsia, blood pressure rises to 140/90 mm Hg (or increases over baseline by 30 mm Hg systolic or 15 mm Hg diastolic), as measured on two occasions at least 6 hours apart. The cause of this rise in blood pressure remains unknown.

Along with elevated blood pressure, many patients with preeclampsia experience proteinuria and edema. Edema generally occurs in the hands and face and

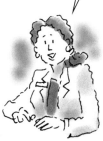

may appear anytime, including after arising in the morning.

Preeclampsia worsening

As preeclampsia worsens, the patient's systolic pressure may be 160 mm Hg or diastolic pressure may be 110 mm Hg, even on bed rest. She may also have:

- altered consciousness
- blurred vision
- epigastric or upper quadrant pain
- hyperreflexia of deep tendon reflexes
- impaired liver function
- oliguria
- thrombocytopenia.

Eclampsia

If not treated effectively, preeclampsia can progress to eclampsia. This condition is marked by signs and symptoms similar to those of preeclampsia but even more severe. Seizures can also occur. Eclampsia may occur before or during labor or within 48 hours after delivery.

> Eclampsia can occur before or during labor or up to 48 hours after delivery.

Treatment

Treat preeclampsia by administering an antihypertensive and by putting the patient on a high-protein diet with normal sodium and fluid intake. It may also help to position the patient laterally, especially on her left side, to avoid compression of the aorta and inferior vena cava.

Treat severe preeclampsia by hospitalizing the patient and by maintaining bed rest in a quiet, darkened room. Administer an antihypertensive and magnesium sulfate, as ordered. If the patient develops eclampsia, implement seizure precautions and administer an anticonvulsant, as ordered.

Quick quiz

1. Ankle edema and jugular vein distention are signs of:

    A. right-sided heart failure.

    B. left-sided heart failure.

    C. CAD.

Answer: A. Right-sided heart failure usually results in a buildup of fluid throughout the body. Look for jugular vein distention, leg and ankle edema, and liver enlargement.

2. The pain of unstable angina usually occurs during periods of:

    A.   exertion.

    B.   marked anxiety.

    C.   little or no exertion.

Answer: C. The pain of unstable angina occurs with little exertion or at rest.

3. In hypertensive retinopathy, damage to retinal blood vessels can cause:

    A.   corneal ulceration.

    B.   swelling of the optic nerve.

    C.   fragmentation of the optic disk.

Answer: B. In hypertensive retinopathy, damage to the blood vessels of the retina can cause blood to leak into the retina and the optic nerve to swell.

Scoring

☆☆☆   If you answered all three questions correctly, great! It's like you've received an I.V. infusion of knowledge!

☆☆   If you answered two questions correctly, terrific! Way to be *un*complicated!

☆   If you answered fewer than two questions correctly, keep cool. Complications get less complicated with each review.

6

Teaching patients with hypertension

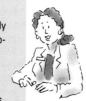

Key facts
◆ Patients with hypertension need to comply with treatment even if they show no symptoms.
◆ Patients can positively affect their own prognosis through lifestyle changes.
◆ A patient who thoroughly understands his antihypertensive therapy is more likely to comply with treatment and avoid adverse reactions.

Teaching strategies

When teaching about hypertension, first explain what blood pressure is and how it's measured. (See *Explaining blood pressure,* page 120.) Explain that many patients with hypertension experience no symptoms of the condition but that treatment remains necessary even so. Tell him that if left untreated, hypertension can damage body organs, including the heart, kidneys, eyes, and brain.

Explaining blood pressure

When teaching about blood pressure, remember to use terms the patient will understand. Tell the patient that blood pressure consists of two numbers. The higher number is a measurement of pressure inside the blood vessels when the heart beats, or contracts. The lower number is a measurement of pressure inside the blood vessels when the heart relaxes between beats. Explain that when the higher number (or systolic pressure) is 140 mm Hg or more or the lower number (or diastolic pressure) is 90 mm Hg or more, the person has high blood pressure.

Control, not cure

Explain that treatment can control but not cure hypertension. By consistently following his treatment regimen, however, the patient can help ensure his own survival and maintain a normal lifestyle.

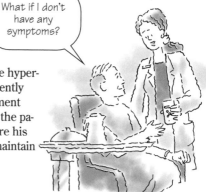

Teaching about the diagnosis

Teach the patient that a diagnosis of hypertension isn't made on the basis of one elevated reading. It requires several readings taken over a period of time. (See *Double-checking a high reading,* page 122.)

Testing hypertension's trail

Explain to the patient that diagnostic tests may be ordered to see if hypertension has led to organ damage. These tests can include:
- urinalysis, to check for renal disease, infection, or diabetes mellitus
- serum potassium level, to check for adrenal gland dysfunction
- blood urea nitrogen or serum creatinine level, to check for renal damage
- renal ultrasound or renal flow scan, to check for renal disease
- chest X-ray, to check for an enlarged heart
- electrocardiogram, to check for heart disease.

Advice from the experts

Double-checking a high reading

When routine blood pressure screening reveals elevated blood pressure in a patient, be sure to:

- check that the cuff size is appropriate for the patient's upper-arm circumference
- take blood pressure readings in both arms
- take readings when the patient is lying, sitting, and standing
- check if the patient smoked, had a caffeine-containing beverage, or felt emotionally upset before the test.

Teaching about lifestyle changes

For patients with mild hypertension, lifestyle modifications form an important element in controlling blood pressure. Discuss with the patient the benefits of exercise, diet changes, and weight reduction.

Exercise

Explain to the patient that any activity, if done daily, can burn calories and help reduce weight. Suggest aerobic exercises, such as walking, jogging, or swimming, and encourage him to choose activities based on his preferences and abilities. (See *Calorie burners*, page 124.)

Advise him to avoid isometric exercises such as weight lifting, which increase workload on the heart and raise blood pressure. Remind him to begin his exercise program gradually and to speak to his primary care provider before beginning.

The patient should do whatever aerobic activity he enjoys, as long as he does it!

Diet

Explain to the patient that there are several modifications he can make in his diet to help reduce blood pressure and improve his overall health. These include:

- reducing salt
- decreasing saturated fat intake
- increasing fiber intake
- reducing alcohol intake.

See ya, sodium

Teach the patient to avoid foods with high sodium content. Also teach him to read the la-

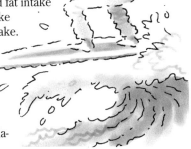

Calorie burners

When counseling your patient about ways to reduce blood pressure, explain the benefits of exercise. Exercise not only strengthens the heart but also burns calories, a must for the patient trying to lose weight. This chart shows the number of calories burned by common activities.

Keep in mind that calorie expenditures may vary considerably, depending on a variety of factors including environmental conditions. Measurements given for adult males are based on a male weighing 175 lb (80 kg) and for adult females, on a female weighing 140 lb (64 kg).

Activity	Calories burned per hour	
	Adult female	Adult male
Light activity Cleaning house Playing baseball Playing golf	240	300
Moderate activity Cycling (5.5 mph) Dancing Gardening Playing basketball Walking briskly (3.5 mph)	370	460
Strenuous activity Jogging (9 minutes/mile) Playing football Swimming	580	730
Very strenuous activity Racquetball Running (7 minutes/mile) Cross-country skiing	740	920

Avoiding high-salt foods

Say no to:
- canned soups
- canned vegetables
- cold cuts
- pickles
- potato chips
- preserved meats.

bels on soft drinks, cereals, and condiments such as ketchup, all of which may contain a large amount of sodium. Advise him to remove the salt shaker from the table and to avoid adding salt to food.

Arrange for dietary counseling for the patient, and have the counselor provide detailed information about the salt content of foods. Ask the counselor to discuss the use of salt substitutes and herbs and spices in cooking.

Forego fat

Teach the patient to decrease the amount of saturated fat in his diet. Explain to him that he should:

• avoid red meat (except for lean cuts) and processed meats, such as cold cuts and hot dogs

• replace whole milk products with low-fat or nonfat milk products

• use olive oil or canola oil in place of saturated tropical oils

• remove the skin from poultry before cooking

• avoid deep-frying

• broil, bake, or poach chicken, turkey, fish, or lean cuts of meat

• eat no more than three egg yolks a week including yolks in prepared foods.

Three egg yolks a week max, including yolks in prepared foods.

Fill in with fiber

Teach the patient to increase his fiber intake. Advise him to eat more dry peas and beans, fruits, pasta, rice, vegetables, and whole grain cereals.

Know your limit

Explain to the patient that too much alcohol may raise his blood pressure. Advise him to limit his daily alcohol intake to less than 24 oz (720 ml) of beer, 9 oz (270 ml) of wine, or 2 oz (60 ml) of hard liquor.

Teaching about drug therapy

A patient with severe hypertension may require drug therapy to control his blood pressure. He'll still need to maintain a heart-healthy lifestyle, however. Explain to the patient that lifestyle modifications can:
- reduce dosage requirements
- enhance beneficial drug effects
- diminish adverse reactions
- help to decrease organ damage as a result of hypertension.

Compliance is the key

Antihypertensives can be effective in controlling hypertension but only when the patient complies with treatment. (See *Drug do's and don'ts at home,* pages 128 and 129.) Studies show that half the patients who begin therapy to control their blood pressure lose contact with their primary care provider within a year.

To encourage compliance, answer all of the patient's or caregiver's questions, and take measures to help him establish an effective home medication routine. (See *Compliance aids,* page 130.) In addition, discuss with the patient the specific anti-

No place like home

Drug do's and don'ts at home

Managing hypertension at home can be a complex process. Patients taking an antihypertensive need to monitor their blood pressure regularly and effectively and be aware of each drug's adverse reactions. Remind the patient to:
• use a self-monitoring blood pressure cuff and to record the reading at least twice weekly in a journal
• take his blood pressure at the same hour each time with the same type of activity preceding the measurement
• report adverse effects to his primary care provider
• avoid high-sodium antacids and over-the-counter (OTC) cold and sinus drugs that may contain a vasoconstrictor (which elevates blood pressure)
• call his primary care provider before taking any OTC drug
• inform his other health care providers about his hypertension and drug therapy.

Smart scheduling

To help your patient develop an effective routine for taking his antihypertensives, you should:
• review each prescription container label with the patient
• determine your patient's normal sleeping patterns, mealtimes, and activities, and work together to schedule the drugs
• prepare a written schedule, listing all drugs, when each should be taken, and whether each should be taken with food or on an empty stomach
• review the completed schedule with the patient and a family member

> **Drug do's and don'ts at home** *(continued)*
>
> • if the patient has a difficult time remembering when to take his anti-
> hypertensive, suggest that he post the schedule in an obvious spot.
>
> **See you soon**
>
> Stress the need for regular follow-up to:
> • monitor blood pressure
> • check laboratory values
> • assess drug therapy
> • evaluate signs and symptoms of organ damage secondary to hyper-
> tension.

hypertensive that he'll be taking and its
adverse reactions.

Vini, vidi, vasodilators

If the patient is taking a vasodilator, explain that the drug lowers blood pressure
by expanding blood vessels. Because vasodilators can lower blood pressure
quickly, teach the patient to monitor his
blood pressure routinely and report low
blood pressure.

Ace ACE inhibitors

If the patient is taking angiotensin-
converting enzyme (ACE) inhibitor, explain that these drugs prevent the body
from retaining sodium and water and

No place like home

Compliance aids

To help a patient comply with oral antihypertensive therapy, measure doses for him using a compliance aid. Because a compliance aid doesn't hold many tablets or capsules, you, the patient, or a caregiver must remember to fill the device regularly.

For today

A 1-day pill pack, a plastic box with four-lidded compartments marked "breakfast," "lunch," "dinner," and "bedtime," can help the patient see whether he has taken all pills prescribed for the day. If needed for a vision-impaired patient, the lids can be embossed with braille characters.

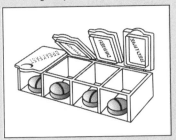

For the week

A 7-day pill pack can help your patient remember whether he has taken the tablets and capsules prescribed for each day of the week. Each box has seven compartments marked with the initials

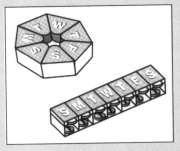

for each day of the week (in both braille characters and printed letters).

thus, lower blood pressure. Teach the patient to:

• watch for dizziness, headache, or fatigue and to report these symptoms to his primary care provider

• report rash, which may indicate hypersensitivity

• monitor his blood pressure regularly

• report chronic, dry, nonproductive cough.

> I'll help you establish a schedule for taking your blood pressure pills.

Angiotensin blocker, the sequel

If the patient is taking an angiotensin II blocker, explain that these drugs also prevent the body from retaining sodium and water and thus, lower blood pressure. Teach the patient to:

• watch for dizziness (See *Orthostatic hypotension with vasodilators,* page 132.)

• monitor blood pressure regularly

• avoid salt substitutes that contain potassium; they may cause hyperkalemia when used with these drugs.

Listen up!

Orthostatic hypotension with vasodilators

While taking vasodilators, the patient may experience orthostatic hypotension. To avoid this reaction, teach him to:
• rise slowly from a lying to a sitting position
• position his feet firmly on the floor before standing up
• sit or lie down immediately if he feels light-headed or dizzy
• report dizziness to his primary care provider
• avoid making sudden or abrupt changes in direction when walking.

Bran for calcium channel blockers

If the patient is taking a calcium channel blocker, explain that the drug lowers blood pressure and reduces heart rate and cardiac output. Teach the patient to:
• monitor his blood pressure regularly
• report signs and symptoms of heart failure, such as peripheral edema and weight gain
• increase fiber to combat constipation, a common adverse reaction.

Diurese, please

If the patient is taking a diuretic, explain that the drug lowers blood pressure by increasing urine output. Encourage the patient to take diuretics early in the day or evening to avoid nocturia. Monitor blood pressure and weight regularly. (See *Potassium pointers,* page 134.)

Adrenergic alert

If the patient is taking an adrenergic blocker, explain that the drug relaxes blood vessel walls and lowers blood pressure. Alert the family or caregiver to watch for adverse reactions, such as drowsiness, depression, or mental confusion. Teach the patient to:
• monitor blood pressure regularly
• monitor weight daily and report significant gains
• report sexual dysfunction such as impotence, a possible adverse reaction.
• change position slowly (if taking an alpha-adrenergic blocker), especially from lying to standing, due to possible orthostatic hypotension
• if another adrenergic blocker is added, be alert for syncope after the initial dose
• watch for and report signs and symptoms of heart failure, such as leg and ankle edema or difficulty breathing, especially at night.

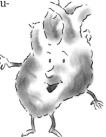

Hellooooo. How 'bout a little bran for breakfast, huh?

Listen up!

Potassium pointers

Certain diuretics can decrease the potassium level in the patient's blood. If the patient is taking a potassium wasting diuretic, tell him to eat foods rich in potassium, such as bananas, orange juice, and tomatoes.

Spare the bananas

However, if the patient is using a potassium sparing diuretic, he should instead restrict foods high in potassium. He should also report:

• symptoms of hypokalemia, such as weakness, muscle cramps, or tremors
• symptoms of ototoxicity, such as hearing changes or ringing in his ears
• constipation, which can be a adverse reaction of diuresis. If constipation results, he should increase his intake of dietary fiber.

Central action

If the patient is taking a centrally acting antiadrenergic, explain that the drug lowers blood pressure by acting on the central nervous system. Teach the patient:

• that abruptly stopping the drug could lead to rebound hypertension
• to monitor blood pressure regularly
• to use good mouth care; dry mouth is an adverse reaction of this drug

Getting connected

Hypertension sites on the Internet

Check these Internet sites for more information on hypertension.

American Heart Association

www.americanheart.org

This excellent site for patients offers links to pages on how to buy and use home blood pressure equipment, what blood pressure levels mean, what dietary guidelines exist, what causes hypertension, what can be done to treat hypertension, and why the condition is unhealthy. Advise your patient to visit this site for basic information.

American Medical Association

www.ama-assn.org

This made-for-the-patient site offers an overview of issues that arise with hypertension, including how high is high, possible effects of hypertension, stopping medication when blood pressure is controlled, the effects of salt on blood pressure, and the effect of weight loss or gain on blood pressure. Your patients will also benefit from a comprehensive breakdown of the various types of drugs for hypertension.

Hypertension Information Center

www.pharminfo.com

This site contains information from various reputable sources, such as the Food and Drug Administration; National Heart, Lung, and Blood Institute; American Society of Hypertension; and others. More suited to health care professionals than patients, visit this site if you need research about hypertension.

Hypertension Network

www.bloodpressure.com

This site provides weekly updates of new research findings and re-

(continued)

Hypertension sites on the Internet *(continued)*

commendations of interest to people with hypertension. All text is written in clear, nontechnical language by primary care providers and nurses who are experts in the field. Tell your patient about this site if he's looking for more sophisticated information about hypertension.

Mayo Clinic
www.mayohealth.org
This site offers an overview of hypertension and guidelines for treatment. Well-crafted charts show the levels of hypertension and treatment options for each level. Visit this site for the latest treatment guidelines from one of the world's foremost health care institutions.

National Institutes of Health
www.nih.gov/health
This site, designed for patients with hypertension, discusses hypertension, diagnostic tests, taking action to control the disease, special concerns for patients with hypertension, menu ideas, exercise ideas, and generic drug names; a glossary is included. Advise your patient to check this site for ideas about exercise and ways to control hypertension.

National Kidney and Urologic Diseases Information Clearinghouse
www.niddk.nih.gov/health/kidney
This site offers information about the connection between kidney disease and hypertension. Check this site if you need data about renal complications of hypertension.

National Library of Medicine
http://medlineplus.nlm.nih.gov/medlineplus
The National Library of Medicine's MEDLINEplus provides links to articles containing information on hypertension. The site also provides a carefully selected list of articles organized by type (reviews, diagnosis, prevention, and treatment). Some articles offer full text; others offer abstracts only. If you're looking for specific information on hypertension, this site is for you.

• taking spironolactone that the drug may initially darken the urine.
• that ice chips, hard candy, or gum can ease dry mouth.

Quick quiz

1. Soft drinks, cereals, and condiments such as ketchup may contain a large amount of:

    A. calcium.
    B. phosphorus.
    C. sodium.

Answer: C. Teach your patient to read the labels on soft drinks, cereals, and condiments such as ketchup, all of which may contain a large amount of sodium.

2. To help prevent hypertension complications, advise your patient to limit his daily alcohol intake to less than:

    A. 24 oz (720 ml) of beer.
    B. 10 oz (300 ml) of wine.
    C. 5 oz (150 ml) of hard liquor.

Answer: A. Advise your patient to limit his daily alcohol intake to less than 24 oz of beer, 9 oz (265 ml) of wine, or 2 oz (60 ml) of hard liquor.

3. If your patient is taking an angiotensin II blocker, explain that the drug acts by:

    A.   relaxing the artery walls.

    B.   blocking the flow of calcium across cell membranes.

    C.   preventing the body from retaining sodium and water.

Answer: C. If the patient is taking an angiotensin II blocker, explain that these drugs prevent the body from retaining sodium and water and thus lower blood pressure.

Scoring

☆☆☆   If you answered all three questions correctly, A+! You've earned your apples as a hypertension teacher!

☆☆   If you answered two questions correctly, all right! You're ready to commandeer the classroom!

☆   If you answered fewer than two questions correctly, it's okay. Multiple readings of this chapter will ensure superior results!

Index

A

Acebutolol, 72t-73t
ACE inhibitors. *See* Angiotensin-converting
    enzyme inhibitors.
Age as risk factor, 26
Aldactone, 89t
Alpha-adrenergic antagonists. *See*
    Alpha-adrenergic blockers.
Alpha-adrenergic blockers, 69t-72t
    teaching patient about, 133
Altace, 65t
Amiloride hydrochloride, 83t-84t
Amlodipine besylate, 78t
Angina as coronary artery disease symptom,
    102
Angiotensin-converting enzyme inhibitors,
    65t-69t
    teaching patient about, 129, 131
Angiotensin II blockers, 65t
    teaching patient about, 131
Antihypertensives
    elderly patient and, 62
    emergency, risks of, 112
Apresoline, 91t-92t
Atenolol, 73t
Atherosclerosis as cause of hypertension,
    10i, 11i
Auscultation in physical examination, 41, 43
Auscultatory gap, 49
Automatic blood pressure monitoring, 52i-53i

B

Baroreceptors, 7
Benazepril hydrochloride, 65t-66t

Beta-adrenergic antagonists. *See*
    Beta-adrenergic blockers.
Beta-adrenergic blockers, 72t-78t
    teaching patient about, 133
Blocadren, 77t-78t
Blood pressure, 5, 9i
    auscultatory gap and, 49
    automatic monitoring of, 52i-53i
    average readings for, 44t
    changes in, during pregnancy, 114-115
    cuff placement for measurement of,
        45-46, 48i
    elements that determine, 5, 6
    in hypertension, 1
    Korotkoff sounds and, 47-49
    measuring, 43-50
        in child, 54, 55i, 56
    patient positioning for measurement of,
        44-45, 46
    recording, 49
    stethoscope placement for measurement
        of, 47, 48i
Blood volume
    blood pressure and, 6
    as cause of hypertension, 12i
Bumetanide, 84t-85t
Bumex, 84t-85t

C

Calan SR, 80t
Calcium channel blockers, 78t-80t
    teaching patient about, 132
Capillary fluid shift, blood pressure and, 8
Capoten, 66t-67t
Captopril, 66t-67t

i refers to an illustration; t refers to a table.

Cardene, 79t-80t
Cardiac complications, 99-103
Cardiac output, blood pressure and, 6
Cardiovascular signs and symptoms, 36
Cardura, 69t-70t
Carteolol, 73t-74t
Cartrol, 73t-74t
Catapres, 81t
Centrally acting antiadrenergics, 80t-83t
    teaching patient about, 134, 137
Central nervous system complications,
        104-106
Cerebrovascular accident
    as hypertension complication, 104-105
    signs and symptoms of, 104
    treatment of, 105
Cerebrovascular signs and symptoms, 36
Chemoreceptors, 8
Children, assessing hypertension in, 51, 54,
        55i, 56-58
Chlorthalidone, 85t
Chlorothiazide, 85t-86t
Clonidine hydrochloride, 81t
Coarctation of the aorta, secondary hyper-
        tension and, 18t
Compliance aids, 130i
Corgard, 75t
Coronary artery disease
    angina as symptom of, 102
    as hypertension complication, 102-103
    treatment of, 102-103
Cozaar, 68t-69t
Cuff placement in blood pressure measure-
        ment, 45-46, 48i
Cushing's syndrome, secondary hyperten-
        sion and, 18t

D

Diabetes mellitus, secondary hypertension
        and, 18t
Diagnostic tests, 50-51
    teaching patient about, 121
Diastolic pressure in hypertension, 1, 3t
Diazoxide, 90t-91t
    as emergency antihypertensive, 112
Diet
    as risk factor, 28-31
    teaching patient about, 123, 125-126
Dissecting aortic aneurysm as hypertension
        complication, 103
Diuretics, 83t-89t
    teaching patient about, 132-133, 134
Diuril, 85t-86t
Doxazosin mesylate, 69t-70t
Drug therapy, 62, 63-95
    angiotensin-converting enzyme
            inhibitors and, 65t-69t
    alpha-adrenergic blockers and, 69t-72t
    beta-adrenergic blockers and, 72t-78t
    calcium channel blockers and, 78t-80t
    centrally acting antiadrenergics and,
            80t-83t
    compliance with, importance of, 127, 129,
            130i
    diuretics and, 83t-89t
    ethnic differences in response to, 95
    home management of, 128-129
    modification of, as treatment step, 63-64
    steps of, 63-64
    teaching patient about, 127-129, 131-134,
            137
    vasodilators and, 90t-93t
DynaCirc, 79t

E

Eclampsia, 116-117
Elderly patient, antihypertensives and, 62
Emergency complications, 108-113
Enalapril maleate, 67t
Encephalopathy, hypertensive, 105
Esidrix, 88t-89t
Esmolol as emergency antihypertensive, 112
Essential hypertension, 2-3
    causes of, 17
Ethacrynate sodium, 86t
Ethnic differences in drug response, 95
Exercise
    lack of, as risk factor, 31-32
    teaching patient about, 122-123, 124t

F

Family history
    patient assessment and, 39
    as risk factor, 26
Fosinopril sodium, 67t-68t
Funduscopic examination, 42i
Furosemide, 87t

G

Gender as risk factor, 26-27
Guanabenz acetate, 82t
Guanfacine hydrochloride, 82t-83t

H

Headaches, hypertension and, 37
Health history, patient assessment and,
    37-40
    for child, 56-58

Heart failure
    as hypertension complication, 99-102
    left-sided, 101
    right-sided, 100-101
    treatment of, 101-102
High blood pressure. *See* Hypertension.
Home management of drug therapy, 128-129
Hormonal regulators, blood pressure and, 8
Hydralazine hydrochloride, 91t-92t
Hydrochlorothiazide, 88t-89t
HydroDIURIL, 88t-89t
Hygroton, 85t
Hyperstat IV, 90t-91t
Hypertension
    assessing
        in adults, 37-51
        in children, 51, 54, 55i, 56-58
    blood pressure in, 1
    causes of, 10i-14i
    classifying, 3t
    complications of, 5, 24-25, 99-117
    definition of, 1-2
    follow-up guidelines for, 94t
    headaches and, 37
    home management of, 128-129
    incidence of, 23, 24
    Internet sites for, 135-136
    patient teaching for, 119-137
    pathophysiology of, 8, 17, 18t-19t, 20
    pregnancy and, 114-117
    prevalence of, 23
    preventing, 23-33
    risk factors for, 25-33
    secondary, 3-5
        causes of, 4-5, 18t-19t
    signs and symptoms of, 36
    sustained, effects of, 15i-16i

i refers to an illustration; t refers to a table.

Hypertension *(continued)*
    treatment of, 57-58, 61-98
    types of, 2-5
Hypertensive crisis, 109-113
    categories of, 109-110
    signs and symptoms of, 110-111
    treatment of, 111-113
Hypertensive encephalopathy, 105
Hypertensive retinopathy, 106
Hytrin, 71t-72t

I-J

Idiopathic hypertension, 2-3
Inderal, 76t-77t
Inspection in physical examination, 40-41
Internet, hypertension sites on, 135-136
Isoptin SR, 80t
Isradipine, 79t

K

Korotkoff's sounds, 47-49

L

Labetalol hydrochloride, 70t
Lasix, 87t
Levatol, 76t
Lifestyle changes
    teaching patient about, 122-126
    as treatment step, 62-63
Loniten, 92t
Lopressor, 74t-75t
Losartan potassium, 68t-69t
Lotensin, 65t-66t

M

Malignant hypertension, 4, 108-109
    signs and symptoms of, 108-109
    treatment of, 109
Medical history, patient assessment and, 39
Metoprolol tartrate, 74t-75t
Midamor, 83t-84t
Minipress, 71t
Minoxidil, 92t
Monopril, 67t-68t
Multidrug therapy as treatment step, 64

N

Nadolol, 75t
Neural regulators, blood pressure and, 7-8
Neurologic disorders, secondary hypertension and, 19t
Nicardipine hydrochloride, 79t-80t
Nitropress, 92t-93t
Nitroprusside sodium, 92t-93t
    as emergency antihypertensive, 112
Normodyne, 70t
Norvasc, 78t

O

Obesity as risk factor, 28
Oretic, 88t-89t

P-Q

Palpation in physical examination, 41
Parathyroid gland dysfunction, secondary hypertension and, 18t
Patient teaching, 119-137
    about blood pressure, 120, 122
    about diagnosis, 121

i refers to an illustration; t refers to a table.

Patient teaching *(continued)*
    about drug therapy, 127-129, 130i, 131-134, 137
    about lifestyle changes, 122-126
    strategies for, 119-120
Pediatric patient, assessing hypertension in, 51, 54, 55i, 56-58
Penbutolol sulfate, 76t
Phentolamine mesylate, 70t
Pheochromocytoma
    secondary hypertension and, 19t
    surgical treatment for, 93-95
Physical examination, 40-41, 42i, 43-50, 44t, 48i, 52i-53i
Pituitary gland dysfunction, secondary hypertension and, 18t
Prazosin hydrochloride, 71t
Preeclampsia, 115-116, 117
Pregnancy
    hypertension and, 114-117
    secondary hypertension and, 19t
Primary aldosteronism, secondary hypertension and, 19t
Propranolol hydrochloride, 76t-77t

R
Race as risk factor, 27
Ramipril, 65t
Regitine, 70t
Renal complications, 106-108
Renal failure
    as hypertension complication, 106-108
    signs and symptoms of, 107
    treatment of, 107-108
Renal parenchymal disease, secondary hypertension and, 19t

Renin-angiotensin-aldosterone system
    blood pressure regulation and, 6, 13i
    changes in, during pregnancy, 114
Renin excretion, excessive, as cause of hypertension, 13i
Renovascular disease, secondary hypertension and, 19t
Retinal examination, 42i
Retinopathy, hypertensive, 106

S
Secondary hypertension, 3-5
    causes of, 4-5, 18t-19t
Sectral, 72t-73t
Single-drug therapy as treatment step, 63
Smoking as risk factor, 32
Social history, patient assessment and, 40
Sodium Edecrin, 86t
Spironolactone, 89t
Stress
    as cause of hypertension, 14i, 32
    techniques to reduce, 32-33
Surgical treatment, 93-95
Systolic pressure in hypertension, 1, 3t

T-U
Tenex, 82t-83t
Tenormin, 73t
Terazosin hydrochloride, 71t-72t
Thyroid gland dysfunction, secondary hypertension and, 18t
Timolol maleate, 77t-78t
Trandate, 70t

i refers to an illustration; t refers to a table.

V

Vascular resistance, blood pressure and, 7
Vasodilators, 90t-93t
     teaching patient about, 129, 131
Vasotec, 67t
Verapamil hydrochloride, 80t
Viscosity of blood as cause of hypertension,
          12i

W-Z

Wytensin, 82t

i refers to an illustration; t refers to a table.